The **ethics of medical research on humans**

One of the most difficult problems that con~~f~~ ..ns and medical professionals is how to apply ethical princip..s t... ... decisions affecting patients. In this even-handed book, Claire Fost.. ..mines the three main approaches to moral decision-making: goal-based, duty-based and right-based. She examines the underlying philosophical arguments of each, their relative strengths and weaknesses, and how they can actually be applied. She also looks at the problematic boundaries where treatment ends and experimentation begins. Is it ethical to experiment with new cures on people who are probably dying anyway? And how do you assess quality of consent? This book provides a thorough, non-partisan grounding in what the ethical principles are and what informs them. It is an invaluable preparation both for a researcher being interviewed by an ethics committee and for the people sitting on the committee, and will be essential reading for all medical decision-makers.

Claire Foster has developed a unique and systematic approach to analysing the ethics of human participant research through her experience running the Research Ethics Committee Project at the King's College Centre of Medical Law and Ethics. She also has extensive experience of training members of research ethics committees and commenting on guidelines drawn up by such bodies as the Medical Research Council, the Royal College of Physicians and the Nuffield Council on Bioethics.

The ethics of medical research on humans

Claire Foster

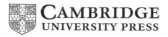

CAMBRIDGE
UNIVERSITY PRESS

PUBLISHED BY THE PRESS SYNDICATE OF THE UNIVERSITY OF CAMBRIDGE
The Pitt Building, Trumpington Street, Cambridge, United Kingdom

CAMBRIDGE UNIVERSITY PRESS
The Edinburgh Building, Cambridge CB2 2RU, UK
40 West 20th Street, New York NY 10011-4211, USA
10 Stamford Road, Oakleigh, VIC 3166, Australia
Ruiz de Alarcón 13, 28014 Madrid, Spain
Dock House, The Waterfront, Cape Town 8001, South Africa

http://www.cambridge.org

First published 2001

Printed in the United Kingdom at the University Press, Cambridge

Typeface Minion 10/12pt   *System* Poltype® [v n]

A catalogue record for this book is available from the British Library

Library of Congress Cataloguing in Publication data

Foster, Claire, 1964–
The ethics of medical research on humans/Claire Foster.
    p.;   cm.
Includes bibliographical references and index.
ISBN 0 521 64196 9 (hardback) – ISBN 0 521 64573 5 (pbk.)
1. Human experimentation in medicine – Moral and ethical aspects.
2. Medicine – Research – Moral and ethical aspects.   3. Medical ethics.   I. Title.
[DNLM: 1. Ethics, Medical.   2. Human Experimentation. W 50 F754e 2001]
R853.H8 F67 2001
174'.28–dc21   2001025216

ISBN 0 521 64196 9 hardback
ISBN 0 521 64573 5 paperback

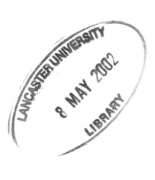

To members of research ethics committees past and present

Contents

Foreword

A few weeks ago I was sitting at my desk, when there was a knock at the door and two characters walked in who bore an uncanny resemblance to two parking meter attendants with whom I had had a mild altercation while parking my car earlier in the day. 'We are carrying out an organ inspection' one of them said, 'we have to look through your office to see if you are hoarding any human tissues or related material'. After they had left, empty handed I hasten to add, I mused on how close we are to Aldous Huxley's *Brave New World* and pondered on the extent to which we, the doctors, have brought all this on ourselves by centuries of insensitivity to the feelings of society.

In the UK, the last few years have seen an endless attack on the medical profession: clinical incompetence; abysmal communication; the storage of children's organs for medical research without permission from their parents; and so much more. All this has brought the inevitable short-term, knee-jerk reactions from Government, and the profession is likely to come under increasingly close scrutiny and bureaucratic regulation. This is happening at a time when we are about to enter one of the most exciting but complex periods of medical research. As the fall-out from the human genome project is applied to clinical research and practice it will open up a whole series of new ethical dilemmas and will undoubtedly raise many new concerns about research on human beings. The more gloomy commentators on the current scene are raising vistas of Nazi Germany, the eugenics movement and the kind of human experimentation that went on in concentration camps under the guise of medical research. Already there are signs of over-reaction, and regulations are being established which will, in the long term, have a deleterious effect on many areas of medical research.

Some good has come from these increasing concerns about the conduct of medical research, however. The Government and the bodies which fund research have become increasingly aware of the importance of the ethical basis of clincal investigation, demanding that young clinical research workers are exposed to instruction in good practice and that all research involving patients is scrutinized more thoroughly by appropriate ethics committees.

The bodies which control medical practice have established their own ethical review processes and this country has taken a valuable lead in establishing an entirely independent body of this type, free of any influence from Government or the medical establishment and industry, the Nuffield Council on Bioethics. Most medical schools are now providing students with courses on ethics at different stages of their training and many universities are establishing departments of bioethics.

While all this activity is commendable, and will undoubtedly do much to restore people's faith in the activities of the medical profession, there is a danger that the simple principles on which the ethical basis of medical research are founded are lost in a mist of political correctness. In this splendid new book, Claire Foster has provided an excellent account of the underlying philosophy on which the ethics of medical research is based. Building on this foundation she has examined some of the major issues which cause so much confused thinking about the ethics of experimentation on humans and, using a series of well chosen examples, has provided sound and commonsense guidelines for medical research workers.

Commendably short and free of the jargon which haunts this field, this introduction to the really important issues of research on humans should provide young clinical research workers with a solid basis on which to develop their programmes, and, at the same time, help to remind established clinical scientists about the central ethical issues which underline this field, and which are so often lost in the complex maze of ill-thought-through responses to new problems which, sadly, typifies the current biomedical research scene.

Claire Foster has done us all a great service in writing this small and extremely clear account of the fundamentals of bioethics as they apply to research on human beings. I wish this book all the success it deserves.

D. J. Weatherall
Oxford, June 2001

Acknowledgements

I would like to thank all those who had a hand in making this book possible. All my teachers played their part in this, but I want to thank Sophie Botros in particular, whose careful imparting to me of her approach to moral philosophy and medical ethics has so influenced this book. I should also like to thank David Lloyd, Laura Wilson, James and Katie Glover and Cyril Chapman for their very helpful comments on earlier drafts. Jo Sumner, Madeleine Barnes and Rebecca Fallon all provided vital support when it was needed, for which grateful thanks are due. Most of all I want to thank David for his unfailing, gentle presence and unselfish support.

An introduction to the ethical issues

Introduction

It must be the dream of any ill person to be cured effectively and immediately, with no side effects. Every doctor's dream must be to provide such a precise service. It might happen sometimes, but the reality is rarely so satisfactory. Even when 'miracle cures' like penicillin are discovered, the appearance of absolute cure with no side effects turns out to be different from the actual experience, sometimes long after the medicine has been discovered. However, it is just as well that throughout the history of medicine, some doctors have never accepted the idea that complete cures are a delusion and stopped looking for them. For if research is not undertaken, medicine would not progress in the remarkable ways that it has. There may not be many complete cures, but there are treatments for numerous conditions that previously would have killed or disabled for life. It has also been established that some treatments are useless or even harmful. The ultimate goal of medical research must be to find complete cures; the more prosaic actual achievements do, nevertheless, help a great deal.

To improve medical care as much as we can, if not to perfect it, means that we have to accept the need for research. Some argue that the real art of medical care is to prevent people falling ill in the first place. Prevention is better than cure, particularly if it does not involve taking drugs. Even to establish what constitutes healthy living requires research, however. In any case, prevention is helpful to those who have not yet succumbed to the effects of unhealthy living, but for those for whom it is too late, treatment is needed. Also, there are many causes of conditions which, not being understood, or being understood but not being controllable, cannot be avoided or changed. Research into causes is needed, and so is research into treatment of the conditions as they present themselves. Whatever the condition or its cause, medical research is needed. What is more, that research is almost always going to take the form of steps on the way to complete cures, rather than reaching the goal in one go. Giant leaps in understanding and treatment are not, by their very nature, planned, as the story of penicillin's discovery demonstrates. Meanwhile, the pedestrian plodding of routine research has to go on. Over time it can show startlingly good results, such as the hard-won 50% improvement in the treatment of childhood leukaemia.

The recognition of the need for careful research, and participation in it, requires sacrifices on the part both of patients and of doctors. Doctors have to recognize that what knowledge they have had imparted to them is not complete, and that there is always more to learn and pass on within their discipline. To learn, doctors have to be ready to question their established practices and beliefs, and to recognize the possibility of really different ways of treating diseases. To pass on research results, doctors have to be able to communicate with their peers. Research means detailed and disciplined work. Research projects have to be planned and carried out, and their results disseminated. Patients, who would far rather not be treated as guinea pigs, have to be encouraged to want to help. Doctors may risk losing patients to colleagues who do not ask them to take part in research programmes. Doctors who do undertake research need to remember that even in the midst of a research project their patients still require their best interests to be served, and that those interests come before the successful completion of a project, should there be a conflict. Enthusiasm for reaching the goals of research should not make doctors view their patient participants merely as 'good clinical material'.

Patients have to recognize that if medical care is to continue to improve then they must play their part too, and allow their treatments to be offered as part of research programmes, if that is the best way to ensure continuing improvement. If research is well designed then their treatment should not be inferior, but they may have to accept that a computer, not a doctor, will allocate the treatment they receive, so that the doctor's bias is factored out and the results of the research are more reliable. Patients have to understand that, if their doctor says that she does not know which is the best treatment for their condition, but that they can participate in a trial to help find out, she is being a better doctor than the one who wrongly claims absolute knowledge, despite the (false) security conveyed by the second sort of doctor. If the doctor then goes on to suggest that her patients participate in a trial to help discover which treatment is best, the patients have to believe that their doctor has not suddenly transformed from a genial do-gooder to a sinister researcher in a white coat who from now on will not consider them as human beings. That is a big step for many people, who shudder at the thought of human subject research. The staff member at King's College, London, who used to serve our lunch when I was running courses called 'The ethics of research on humans', said as much. 'I saw the posters for your course,' she told me. 'It looks *horrible.*'

Such gut reactions are probably typical. They reflect the perception that being a good and caring doctor and being a good researcher simultaneously is not possible. They also indicate a lack of understanding of the need for medical research to underpin good doctoring. But the King's College staff member could be the next patient in hospital eligible for enrolment in a research project. If her autonomy is to be respected, she is going to need to be fairly persuaded that the research is worth doing, and can be done in an ethical way.

This book is not written for the staff member, but the concerns that lie behind her shudder are where the ethics of research on humans are located. So although some might argue that medical research needs no justification, I would like to consider first of all the reasons why medical research has to be undertaken, and then go on to the question of how it can be done ethically.

What is the value of research?

Those who support the need for research argue that no new treatment should be offered outside the context of a controlled trial, so that the treatment's effectiveness and efficacy can be measured *ab initio*, not only for the sake of the patient receiving it but also for future patients. This view entails that patients should by custom and practice also be experimental subjects. Few would rather be a guinea pig than the recipient of tried and tested treatment, but the proponents of clinical trials point out that even an established treatment which is given outside the context of a trial is more often than not untested and unproven. Hence patients receiving it are, *de facto* if not *de jure*, guinea pigs in a uncontrolled trial whose outcomes are not being measured consistently.

Baum (1986) explained that the surgeon who carries out mastectomy for early breast cancer for 10 years and then switches to lumpectomy for the next 10 years, because custom and practice have changed, is in fact conducting a research project involving 'haphazard allocation'. The surgeon's patients are not receiving the best known treatment, they are receiving the treatment that she thinks is best on the basis of unreliable data. Because the surgeon is acting solely in what she believes to be the best interests of her patients, and her intentions towards them are unmixed with the desire to gain knowledge which will not be of direct benefit to them, the ethics of her behaviour have not, in the past, been openly questioned.

On the other hand, the surgeon might undertake a properly designed controlled trial, in which half her patients were chosen randomly (a technical word which means that patients' treatment is determined by the equivalent of tossing a coin rather than anyone's deliberate choice) to receive mastectomy and half to receive lumpectomy. If she then compared the treatment outcomes for each group, she would produce objectively convincing evidence for which of the two treatments is the better, instead of continuing in uncertainty or, worse still, thinking she knew which was better when she did not.

Whilst few would deny the need to demonstrate greater certainty than subjective observation allows, the attitude of the surgeon to the individual patients in the trial might nevertheless then be open to rebuke, because arguably she is not doing her best for each one, but treating each as a means to her own end: that of answering the question of whether mastectomy or lumpectomy is the better treatment for early breast cancer. However, Baum would argue that in fact the surgeon *is* doing the best for each of her patients because she is offering a 50% chance of receiving the best treatment, *whichever it is*. Since she does not know for certain which is better, it would be wrong for her to offer treatment in any other way than randomly (understood in its technical sense). If she switched to lumpectomy, without finding out for certain whether it was the better treatment, she might be exposing her patients to unknown risks and uncertain benefits. Hence, for the surgeon, putting her patients into such a trial means they are better off than if she offered just one of the two treatments.

The treatment for childhood leukaemia and the side effects of diethylstyl-boesterol are examples of why research is so important. For some decades in the UK, research into treatments for childhood leukaemia has been organized nationally, so that most children presenting with leukaemia will (with their parents' consent) be randomly allocated either the latest proven treatment or the latest novel and experimental treatment. As a result of this collaborative and carefully orchestrated activity, treatment for leukaemia has moved from being mostly unsuccessful to being 50% successful, in that mortality from the condition has dropped from 100% to 50%. The story of treatment development for leukaemia is an astounding success, from the point of view of its consequences. It has not been the result of some single, radical discovery like that of penicillin, which brought about a complete shift in the paradigm of treatment of those diseases which antibiotics can cure. Rather, it took, and continues to take, painstakingly small steps that have inched forward over years. Had such careful research not been conducted, successful treatments for leukaemia may have been developed, but, as Baum would argue, the discoveries would have been haphazard, subject to chance, and unlikely to have been received into the generality of practice so readily, since their efficacy would not be proven in the eyes of others.

Diethylstyboesterol was first synthesized in 1938 and administered to several million pregnant women to prevent spontaneous abortion and premature delivery (Dodds et al., 1938). Much later, in the 1970s, a group of doctors noticed a connection between the mother's exposure to the drug and the likelihood of her child, if female, contracting vaginal cancer (Noller and Fish, 1974). Now there are indications that the cancer risk is not so great as the 1970s observations indicated (Hatch et al., 1998). If the drug had been introduced by means of a properly conducted randomized controlled trial, with follow up of the patients in the trial, the questions about cancer would have been discovered by the 1940s or 1950s at the latest. Because the drug was administered in an uncontrolled fashion, risks were only noticed much later on by chance observation and linking of factors in the women concerned, and even then they were not properly quantified.

What are the limitations of research?

Black warns against a 'total surrender to the scepticism that is theoretically demanded by the scientist' (1998). Some aspects of medicine are inappropriate for the researcher to question. Black argues that although there is a growing minority of situations in which scientific medicine 'makes all the difference between a cure and a disaster ... we should keep in mind that they are still, however important, only a small part of the whole province of medicine, and that we have a "duty of care" as well as a "duty of cure"'. He quotes Robert Platt:

However far the science of medicine and of surgery advances, the art of medicine will remain: the art of first identifying the patient's problem (which is something more than merely diagnosing his disease) and the art of applying the science to the need of the individual patient. (Platt, 1972, p. 27)

Imagine a patient who presents his medical problem to his doctor, and asks her to do what is best for him. This doctor is persuaded of the reliability and desirability of randomized controlled trials. Armed with data, she explains the treatment options for her patient's condition, their probable success rate and the statistical likelihood of unwanted side effects. However, the patient, instead of considering in a scientific way the relative merits of the options in front of him, repeats his question, asking the doctor to do what *she* believes is best for him. The patient trusts in and wants his doctor's feelings and intuitions about himself in particular, not numbers and risk percentages for people who are like but not him. The doctor, unless she has trained herself to be mechanical in her response to her patients, is unlikely not to have such feelings and intuitions. Now the proponent of the randomized controlled trial will argue that unless knowledge is generated from the controlled situation of a trial, it is unreliable and should be ignored. This view underestimates what Black would call the ability and tendency of clinicians to work on a balance of probabilities, to which I would add their capacity for responding in detail to precisely what is in front of them. There are all sorts of differences between patients that may have important implications for the kinds of treatments they should receive. These differences may or may not be commensurable. The controlled trial may be capable of counting them in, or it may need to factor them out by means, *inter alia*, of randomization and sample size. Other kinds of research methods may be employed to measure the less quantifiable aspects of the medical encounter, and these will be discussed elsewhere. But the fact remains that nothing can replicate precisely *this* encounter. Hence, the doctor in the example *should* bring her intelligence, intuition and experience to the particular patient in front of her.

It would be reasonable to combine both the science of medicine and the art of it as 'interwoven activities' (Black, 1998). Doctors need to know what research has discovered and then apply it to individual cases as they think fit, trusting in their intuitive responses, but also testing them against good empirical data to ensure they have not wandered off track in any way. Good doctors would be expected to know the relevant data gathered from well-designed, reliable research, and also to respond fully to the individual patients in front of them.

Of course, if doctors are to use data which are reliable, the research which generates them needs to be scientifically sound. There are a number of problems with this, and numerous possible solutions, because different research questions need appropriate methods for answering them. Finding out whether a particular drug lowers patients' blood pressure will require one kind of method; finding out how the drug affects patients' quality of life will require another. Debates persist over the extent to which different research designs are capable of producing reliable answers. Some designs rely heavily on subjective interpretation, for example. This sort of method is regarded with suspicion by many doctors. The issue is significant because the purpose of research is to produce data that are widely accepted. If a doctor goes to the trouble of conducting a research project whose results are disregarded because nobody thinks the study was properly designed, her endeavour, and all the resources it used, is wasted.

What is the right way to treat human research participants?

Dealing with such scientifically thorny questions as what constitutes reliable evidence would be difficult enough if the research subjects were, say, plants. But they are human beings, often patients, who must be treated with due respect. I have already moved away from the theoretically simple perspective of Baum and others, in which, provided there is genuine uncertainty about different treatments, the most appropriate treatment for a patient would be that which was allocated to him within a clinical trial. For, if doctors' proper care of their patients consists of more than a machine-like response to symptoms, then more will be required of them than just to be in a state of uncertainty about treatments before routinely offering them as part of a randomized controlled trial. Their duty of care includes taking into account each individual patient, towards whom, as I have suggested, doctors will have quite specific responses, inappropriate to blind allocation of treatment. It is the suggestion that the controlled trial removes this latter aspect of the doctor's duty of care that gives people in general a feeling of discomfort about, or even fear of, the notion of being research participants or of doctors being researchers, using their patients as their guinea pigs. It can be argued that by comparison with what is on offer outside the context of a clinical trial, being a participant in a trial is by far the preferable option (Chalmers, 1994). But that does not make the fact of becoming a statistic rather than being recognized as an individual any more desirable.

The problem is made more acute by the observation that the scientific validity of the trial, that is, its capacity to yield reliable results, *depends* upon a mechanical method of allocating treatments. In recognition of precisely this natural tendency of doctors to have specific responses to individual patients, the process of random allocation of treatments within trials has been made 'doctor-proof'. It used to be the case that doctors participating in research would be given a series of sealed envelopes, and asked to open them in turn as each patient presented for treatment within the trial. The envelopes would contain instructions as to which treatment should be offered, and the envelopes were randomized. Doctors would, notoriously, open the next envelope for the next patient, decide that it was not the best treatment for this patient, and keep on opening envelopes until the treatment instructions inside accorded with their idea of what this particular patient needed. Most randomized controlled trials now use a computer to allocate treatment, and participating doctors will be required to telephone a study centre as each patient in the trial presents, to be told by a computer which is the treatment to be allocated. For one of the purposes of random allocation is to erase all possibility of the results of the research being arrived at by virtue of a doctor's bias. But which patient is going to be happy for a computer to 'choose' his treatment rather than a doctor? A qualitative study of parents of children in the national extra corporeal membrane oxygenation (ECMO) study found this attitude amongst parents interviewed:

They [the parents] said they could not understand how a decision could be based on only a name, but also had problems when they considered the possibility that the computer had the information about their daughter's case. To them, she clearly needed treatment other than the conventional care she was receiving and with her details to hand it was incomprehensible that she was not given ECMO. They felt the computer had made the wrong decision. (Snowdon *et al.*, 1997)

It could be argued that the patients' feelings about how treatments are allocated in a trial can be set aside if the doctors are satisfied that the method works in the best interests of their patients. If a doctor is for any reason unhappy for her patient to be randomly allocated a treatment then the patient should not be invited to enter the trial. Hence, the problems with blind allocation might only be found within patient perceptions and not in reality. The problem would therefore be solved by better communication with patients. That doctors are clear in their own minds about when patients are eligible for either treatment and therefore for the trial is belied by the envelope problem. However, this too may be an issue to do with doctors' misperceptions in that they too may believe wrongly in the efficacy of a particular treatment, or its benefit for a particular patient.

These observations hang upon certain assumptions about the objective reality of treatment success and the part that attitudes and beliefs of both doctors and patients have to play in the healing process. Randomized controlled trials have been useful because they can factor out both doctors' and patients' attitudes and beliefs. Because of random allocation, it does not matter whether the patient or the doctor believes the treatment will work. It will work objectively, or not at all. The question then remains whether successful medicine is dependent only on objective factors, or whether beliefs play their part as well, or, even, whether the willingness to accept objective factors depends upon prior beliefs. For example, is it necessary that a patient should have faith in his doctor for the doctor to be able to help him at all? At a minimum level the answer must be yes, because why otherwise would her patient seek and then act upon her advice? Suppose, then, that research was able to establish objectively that some medicines were better than others, but that in the process of establishing that fact – in the process of research – patients lost their faith in the medical profession because of the constant use of computers to allocate treatment?

Arguably, then, there is a dilemma: while the results of research are needed because they should form part of any good doctor's decision-making process, the means by which that information is obtained presents ethical problems. Although it is possible to show that the treatments offered within a controlled trial are the best available, what is lost is the individualized care, which was described earlier as an essential complement to the scientifically supported knowledge of appropriate treatments.

How can research participants' views be respected?

The case is made more complicated if it is considered that the ideal, individualized encounter between patients and doctors ought to include due consideration, not only of each patient's clinical condition, but also of his own thoughts, feelings, concerns and beliefs about both the condition and the proposed treatment. Random treatment allocation ensures that patient bias as well as doctor bias is factored out as a cause of the results of the research, since by the same 'coin-tossing' chance the patient's views on which is the treatment of choice are discounted.

Perhaps, however, instead of complicating the matter further, the introduction of the wishes and needs of individual patients is a way out of this *impasse* between the scientific need to generate unbiased data, and the doctor's duty to respond sensitively to each individual. Suppose that patients actively wish to participate in research? Provided that their wish is based upon adequate information and is freely made, it could be argued that doctors then have no right to override them. The matter becomes one of patients' right to self-determination; doctors need only ensure that the patients have sufficient information and then leave them to make their own decisions. If the problem of the ethical acceptability of research is shifted on to the shoulders of the research subject, I have, arguably, retained the individually tailored response, since it is precisely an individual choice whether or not to take part.

However, by suggesting that the ethical question is answered by passing it on to the patient, the issue has been fudged. All the patient is agreeing to is treatment allocation by chance, which, after all, is all that the doctor was accepting. The individual choice of a particular treatment is still not being made. Moreover, there is always the danger that patients will agree, not because they think it is the right choice, but because their doctor has asked them, and they believe their doctor has their best interests at heart. The extent to which the patients' consent could be called an *informed* choice is, therefore, brought into question. Again, we are faced with the possibility that conducting research on humans is unethical, this time on the grounds that the right of individuals to self-determination is not being honoured. Arguably, then, research has not only brought into question the doctor's duty of care, but also the validity of patient consent.

Three areas of ethical concern in research: science, best interests and autonomy

In the foregoing discussion of the sorts of moral concerns that issue from research on humans, three broad areas have been looked at. The first is in the realm of what is necessary or valuable research, in terms both of its goals and of whether its methods will achieve the goals reliably. The second area concerns the doctor's moral obligation to do the best for her patients, understanding that to be not merely producing a textbook response but tailoring treatments to particular individuals. The third area lies in the realm of considering the wishes and needs of patients and potential research participants, who have rationality to be respected and benefits to gain or lose by virtue of their participation in research, about which only they may know.

These are the three areas on which the ethics of a research project will hinge. Therefore, if we want to be able to tell whether any given research project is ethical or not, we need to be able to analyse it by reference to these concerns. In order to do that rigorously, we have to understand why these are the relevant areas of concern, so that we can have confidence in our conclusions. For the same reason, we also need to know how to conduct the analysis.

The three areas of concern about research on humans relate to three important moral theories. The concern with the scientific validity of a research project is related to morality which is teleological (from the Greek *telos*, meaning 'end, purpose'). That is to say, it is predicated on the notion that an action is justified by its results. The second concern, which is about the duty to care for a research subject's welfare, is related to one kind of deontological moral theory (from the Greek *deon -ontos*, meaning 'to be necessary'), which states that the moral agent owes people duties. The third area, concerned with the research subject's autonomy, is related to another kind of deontological theory, which states that the moral agent must respect people's right to self-determination.

Now some would propose that only one of these theories is necessary to make moral decisions. It could be argued, for example, that all that is necessary to decide whether an action is morally right is that its consequences maximize happiness. Or one might decide that all that is needed is to obey some sound principles of duty. Or one might think that, as long as my actions accord with the wishes of those most affected by those actions, then they are morally acceptable. But we have already discovered that the moral questions which arise in the context of research call upon all three of these theories. This means that they all have to be taken seriously, and we have to be able to make them work in combination, or know what to do if they come into conflict.

I therefore propose to investigate each of the moral approaches in turn as they have been described by different moral philosophers. We will find that if we try to make any one of them a comprehensive moral ideal, it will fall short. Taken in combination with the two others, however, a more robust way of making moral decisions emerges. But in so doing, it is necessary to distil from each approach that in it which is useful for the purpose of analysing the ethics of research on humans. I have given my distillation of the three approaches titles which are borrowed from Ronald Dworkin (1977, pp. 168–77), who used them in respect of political philosophy. The titles were successfully adapted to moral philosophy and medical ethics by Sophie Botros, who also applied them to the ethics of research on humans (Botros, 1992).

(i) **The goal-based approach, also known as consequentialism.** Moral theories which work from this perspective judge an action's moral worth by its predicted or actual outcome. The goal at which the action is aimed provides the moral determinant for the action itself. No consideration is given to the question of whether the contents of the action are morally right. Absolute consequentialism is inappropriate for ethical research, but concern with the validity and importance of the research question, that is, its goals, is appropriate. I will call this part of the ethical enquiry *goal-based morality.*

(ii) **The duty-based deontological approach.** Moral theories based on notions of duty proffer rules of conduct related not to the goals at which actions are directed, but to the nature of the actions themselves. An example of such rules is the Ten Commandments (Exodus 20.1ff). The moral justification for people's actions is determined by the extent to which they adhere to the rules. Duty-based deontological theories have weaknesses, but they provide a counter-balance to goal-based arguments that can sometimes be compelling. In considering the ethics of research, the duty-based issues arise in relation to the way the research is conducted, rather than what it is trying to achieve. Rules such as not harming the research participant will apply. These sorts of considerations can be called *duty-based morality.*

(iii) **Right-based deontological moral thinking.** There are many theories of rights, and the language of rights has become common in medical ethics as a counterbalance to overly paternalistic notions of the doctor's duty. For our purposes, the right with which those who conduct research on humans should be concerned is the right to self-determination, or autonomy. Its practical application is to ensure that research participants' consent is sought and their confidentiality respected. This approach can be called *right-based morality.*

This series of moral approaches will provide three distinct perspectives from which to consider the ethics of research, which we will need to be able to combine, for, in practice, every research project will need to be investigated in the light of all three. The combination should produce a systematic approach to deciding what makes research ethical. It should also produce conflict, in that it is not always possible to give equal weight to all three. What to decide in those circumstances is the principal challenge of the ethics of medical research on humans, and forms the basis for the idea that some research is simply unethical. Separating out the different parts of the ethical assessment should make it easier to establish which moral concerns need to take precedence in individual research proposals.

Identifying these moral perspectives, and showing how to use them in the context of research, will hopefully be of assistance in your own moral thinking about research. The issue to be addressed is, ultimately, whether any research project is ethical or not. But if it is to be addressed in a sound and reasonable way, then a prior question has to be answered, which is: What must I take into account if I am to come to a proper decision about whether this research is ethical? This book should provide you with the answers to the latter question, so that you can answer the former yourself.

2

Goal-based morality: scientific rigour in research

The foundations of goal-based thinking

Research should aim to maximize health and minimize harm

A major issue to consider, if we want to know whether a research project involving human subjects is ethical or not, is what the research is aiming to achieve. If its outcomes are useful to medicine in that they maximize health whilst minimizing any harm, and the research is capable of achieving those outcomes, then, it could be argued, it is morally obligatory that it is undertaken.

The philosophical idea that underpins this argument is that the proper aim of humankind is to maximize happiness. The idea's classical formulation is known as utilitarianism. This is an approach to decision-making that has a place by right in our consideration of research, since research is about seeking and finding goals, or outcomes. Hence it is important to understand the implications of trying to maximize happiness. In what follows we will consider this approach to moral thinking, and discuss its origins, strengths and weaknesses. In so doing we will see in which ways the approach can be genuinely useful to the ethics of research, and in which ways detrimental.

Utilitarianism's strengths and weaknesses

Utilitarianism is a method of moral thinking which considers an action's consequences to be the determinant of whether the action itself is right or not. This method was first applied to practical problems by Jeremy Bentham (1748–1832). The foundation principle that Bentham described, and upon which he built his moral philosophy, is this:

1. Nature has placed mankind under the governance of two sovereign masters, *pain* and *pleasure*. It is for them alone to point out what we ought to do, as well as to determine what we shall do. On the one hand the standard of right and wrong, on the other the chain of causes and effects, are fastened to their throne. They govern us in all we do, in all we say, in all we think: every effort we can make to throw off our subjection, will serve but to demonstrate and confirm it. In words a man may pretend to abjure their empire: but in reality he will remain subject to it all the

while. The *principle of utility* recognises this subjection, and assumes it for the foundation of that system, the object of which is to rear the fabric of felicity by the hands of reason and of law. Systems which attempt to question it, deal in sounds instead of senses, in caprice instead of reason, in darkness instead of light.
But enough of such metaphor and declamation: it is not by such means that moral science is to be improved.

2. The principle of utility is the foundation of the present work: it will be proper therefore at the outset to give an explicit and determinate account of what is meant by it. By the principle of utility is meant that principle which approves or disapproves of every action whatsoever, according to the tendency which it appears to have to augment or diminish the happiness of the party whose interest is in question: or, what is the same thing in other words, to promote or to oppose that happiness. I say of every action whatsoever; and therefore not only of every action of a private individual, but of every measure of government.

3. By utility is meant that property in any object, whereby it tends to produce benefit, advantage, pleasure, good, or happiness, (all this in the present case comes to the same thing) or (what comes again to the same thing) to prevent the happening of mischief, pain, evil, or unhappiness to the party whose interest is considered: if that party be the community in general, then the happiness of the community: if a particular individual, then the happiness of that individual. (Bentham, 1789, pp. 33–34)

For Bentham, to determine whether actions are morally right, that is, whether they honour the principle of utility, is a matter of simple mathematics. We have to identify and count the number of individuals affected by our actions, calculate for each person whether the action would increase or decrease his/her happiness, count up how many individuals would be made happy and how many made unhappy, and then act accordingly. Bentham listed what needed to be taken into account when calculating levels of pleasure and pain, namely, their intensity, duration, certainty, propinquity, fecundity and purity. Bentham also stated that calculations should be based upon each person counting as one and no more than one. There were no gradations of importance for different people.

Utilitarianism is appealing: it requires no religious faith, no explicit moral code, no general agreement of what rules must be obeyed, and only one law of nature to accept, which is that everyone wants to experience pleasure and avoid pain. Utilitarianism has been called a minimum commitment morality, for to adopt it we need learn no detailed and demanding moral teaching. We must want to act responsibly, but that is all. In an age of secular rationalism, utilitarianism provides a common morality which does not ask us to acknowledge God.

It could be argued that, as utilitarianism only considers consequences and not the contents of actions, it could allow us to commit morally abhorrent acts, providing that our actions maximize happiness overall. In response to this, utilitarian thinkers after Bentham have suggested that a more sophisticated calculation be performed. Rather than working out which is the morally right action in each case, we have to work out which are the morally desirable rules which we should apply to our actions, according to the utilitarian criterion that they must lead to the greatest happiness for the greatest number. For the purpose of distinguishing the two forms, Bentham's utilitarianism has been called 'act utilitarianism', and this more sophisticated form has been called 'rule utilitarianism'.

The trouble with the compromise rule utilitarianism offers is that by means of it the simple and neutral grounds for calculation are lost. For rule utilitarianism requires, first, the identification of those rules which we believe would lead to the greatest happiness, and, then, to show that they do, in fact, lead to the greatest happiness. The rules we identify will depend, inevitably, upon what we believe *a priori* to be right. Bentham claimed that no beliefs of any sort are required for moral decisions to be made: all we have to do is to calculate whether our proposed actions will maximize happiness. The circumstances are given and real. For rule utilitarianism, the circumstances are assumed and hypothetical. The realm into which we would reach for rules to set the conditions for the greatest happiness of the greatest number will be the realm of our own ideas and values, there by virtue of (at least) our upbringing and personal experiences. How else did we form the idea that some actions justified by act utilitarianism are morally abhorrent? Rules may, of course, be selected as a result of observation and accumulation of actual consequences of relevantly similar actions over a period of time. But such a selection is still subject to the vagaries of an individual's interpretation. The utilitarian thinker, R.M. Hare, argues that the Love Commandment ('Love the Lord thy God with all thy heart, and with all thy soul, and with all thy mind . . . and love thy neighbour as thyself' Matthew 22.37,39) is the rule which should govern people's actions, because it will maximize happiness (Hare, 1986). Other rule utilitarians identify other rules. Bernard Williams (1993, p. 82ff) argues that utilitarianism, by adopting rules, has retreated into the realm of received tradition and values of which it claimed it had no need.

The cases where a proposed action is justified by act utilitarianism, but is also morally abhorrent, are the cases to which rule utilitarianism may be applied. These are, Williams points out, the very cases that should be supported in order to be a consistent utilitarian, since they are already justified on utilitarian grounds. To take a step back into the realm of rules in order to avoid a morally abhorrent act is inconsistent, since one is supposed to be unaffected by the violation of rules which come from tradition or religion. If an action will maximize happiness, then one should be prepared to perform it, whatever it involves.

If this method of thinking were to be applied to medical research on humans, we would find that a research project has utilitarian moral justification if (i) it is likely to achieve results which can be translated into better medical care for patients; and (ii) the number of research participants is fewer than the number of future beneficiaries; *or* (iii) that the benefit to future patients is of more magnitude than the harm to the research participants, if the number of participants is greater. Chapter One mentioned the leukaemia trials which have led to significant improvements in healthcare. Bentham's criterion of increasing pleasure (good health) or decreasing pain (curing disease or desisting from harmful treatments) is clearly met in the example. The argument could be taken a step further to postulate that the need for such research was and is paramount, and not morally optional. Without it and research like it, medicine would remain in the dark ages, probably doing more harm than good.

However, if that argument is accepted with no deontological qualification, we are also implicitly accepting that it is positively ethical to harm some people for the sake of others. For if an action is performed that does this, we can claim not only that the action was morally right, but that it was morally required, because it maximized happiness. Not performing the action would have minimized happiness. In the case of the leukaemia trials, utilitarianism on its own would require those trials to be conducted *even if* some of the children in the trials were disbenefited, provided that the overall goal was a success, in that treatment for childhood leukaemia in general improved.

In their defence at the Nuremberg Trials, the Nazi doctors used utilitarian arguments to justify their experiments:

Out of 724 experimental persons, 154 died [in the typhus experiments]. But these 154 deaths have to be compared with the 15,000 who died of typhus every day in the camps for Soviet prisoners of war, and the innumerable deaths from typhus among the civilian population of the occupied eastern territories and the German troops. This enormous number of deaths led to the absolute necessity of having effective vaccines against typhus in sufficient quantity. (From the Nazi doctors' defence speeches at the Nuremberg Trials, 1947 p. 1017)

The quotation shows what actions utilitarian-style arguments can be employed to justify. There is nothing in utilitarianism as such to prevent acts which our intuition (or conscience or moral values) would regard as abhorrent. So utilitarianism would not forbid research which harmed its participants, providing its outcome led to more benefit overall.

This is the point where a utilitarian thinker would argue that rule utilitarianism should be adopted. Setting aside Williams' logical quibbles with this version of the theory for the moment, a utilitarian rule which goes like this could be devised: research will be conducted which leads to better medical care, but only if it does not harm the research participants. For this rule to work under utilitarianism, it has to be justified not by any intuitive notion of its being 'simply right', but according to the principle of utility; that is, its application has itself to maximize happiness. Now, it could be argued that no-one would be happy to benefit from research which has harmed others, and on that basis this rule has utilitarian justification. But how do we know that that is the case? In theory, people might agree with the principle, but in practice, if someone has a very ill close relative, would she reject a treatment which might help her relative, but which had also been developed through harming someone else? If she was happy to accept such a treatment, the rule has failed its utilitarian test, and our moral thinking collapses back into act utilitarianism. If the research which harmed some was already justified according to act utilitarianism, and we are thoroughgoing utilitarians, not harbouring latent deontological notions of what is or is not morally acceptable, we should simply agree to the harm.

Williams made a telling observation of the inherent debasing pull of utilitarian philosophy when he said that, being by nature pre-emptive, it is subject to a kind of Gresham's Law (an observation in economics that money of a lower intrinsic value has a tendency to circulate more freely than money of a higher intrinsic and equal nominal value). As Williams puts it:

> There is a simple reason for this: a utilitarian must always be justified in doing the least bad thing which is necessary to prevent the worst thing that would otherwise happen in the circumstances ... – and what he is thus justified in doing may often be something which, taken in itself, is fairly nasty. (Williams, 1993, p. 96)

An example of this kind of thinking is what happens if someone decides to have an abortion. No one would argue that to have an abortion is in and of itself a good action. It could only be found 'good' in the sense that, in that person's mind anyway, not to have an abortion would lead to worse consequences than having an abortion. Similarly, and with apologies for the somewhat insensitive comparison, the Nazi doctors did not try to show that what they had done to their experimental subjects was intrinsically good, but rather they tried to show that under the circumstances their research had to happen, because the consequences of it not happening were much worse.

Goal-based moral thinking applied to medical research

Utilitarianism has the advantage of simplicity in that it only considers the outcome of actions to matter morally. Inherent in this approach is the disadvantage that it can justify or even require harm to some. Hence, utilitarianism fails to offer a sufficient moral basis for considering whether any given research project involving human subjects is morally acceptable or not. For research on humans to be ethical, not only must the consequences of the research be considered, but what procedures and risks the research subjects will be exposed to, and whether the subjects will want to be so used must also be thought about. Utilitarianism cannot help us with these concerns.

However, to dismiss utilitarianism would be to lose an important aspect of moral thinking, which is that we should consider the consequences of our actions before embarking on them. Although consequences should not be regarded as our final, and certainly not our only, justification for deciding whether the action itself is ethical, neither should we ignore them. This is as true for research projects as it is for any other action. Hence, part of our consideration of the ethics of research on humans is to identify what the goal of the research is, and to judge whether it is morally right, not in order to justify bad actions to achieve it, but because it is wrong to commence a research project which has morally questionable aims. This, then, is how we will use utilitarianism. It is a distinctly different version of the usual theory, because it will accept an intuitive notion, that some consequences are 'simply wrong' or, to put it another way, that some sorts of happiness are better than others, and because it will not accept that maximizing happiness is the moral trump card. I call this version 'goal-based morality'.

When this approach to moral thinking is brought to the ethics of research on humans, we are, in effect, asking what use the research results will be to medicine. This concern with the medical or scientific value of research also obliges us to think about two other related issues. These are, first, that the research should be designed in such a way that the goals are achieved satisfactorily, and second, that when they are achieved, they should be disseminated. In a sense, these are technical questions, not ethical ones. But they have serious ethical implications. Badly designed research gives rise to inaccurate results which mislead and are potentially dangerous to patients. Unpublished results, however accurate, help no one except the researcher. The rest of this chapter will address these three areas of moral concern which fall under the heading of goal-based issues.

The application of goal-based thinking

The goals of research

Immediate goals and general directions
In considering what value a research proposal will be to medicine, we find we can judge it in terms of both its immediate goals and the general direction of which the individual project is a part. The immediate goal will present itself as a question, such as: whether or not treatment A works safely and efficiently; whether treatment B restores the balance of all the body's functions; whether situation C is the cause of condition D; whether patients prefer E to F.

These research questions are asked within larger contexts than their immediate aims: within their own therapeutic field; within the field of medicine and healthcare generally; within the direction of human endeavour; and within the environment of the whole world. At each level, questions can be asked about whether the research will have beneficial effects. For example, at the level of the environment, the over-use of pharmaceuticals has had effects which potentially harm everyone, such as the presence of oestrogen in the water supplies, or the growing resistance to antibiotics in populations.

Judging the morality of the goals of research proposals

These general directions to which individual projects contribute raise moral questions, but they cannot be addressed at the level of the individual research project, since it is collectively and cumulatively that they cause problems. If I sit on a research ethics committee and consider a particular research project, I can express qualms about the developments in medicine of which it is a part, but I cannot really justify withholding ethical approval on those grounds alone, for it would seem unfair to load the responsibility for the general problem on to that one project. Moreover, judging the moral desirability of the goal of any research proposal presents problems of what criteria it should be judged against. The goals of maximizing health care whilst minimizing harm can be retained as the ultimate aim, and some research will be clearly moving in that direction. Other research proposals may not be capable of being linked in the same way, and may seem trivial by comparison. They may not be. Even with appropriate expertise amongst their membership, research ethics committees may not understand the contribution of a particular research proposal within the context of the development of the discipline of which it is a part. Hence, it is difficult for research ethics committees to disapprove of a research project on the grounds of its goals alone. The researcher will be in the best position to judge this, though even he may not necessarily know where a particular investigation will lead. He is, nevertheless, morally obliged to consider the ethics of what he is proposing to do, in general as well as in local terms.

Although it is hard to see how a research proposal could be found unethical on its goals alone (unless the goal is manifestly bad, such as developing biological weapons of mass destruction, in which case it will not be conducted in the context of medicine), it still matters that some view is taken of the degree of importance of a proposal's goals. This is partly because the relative importance will make a difference to the view that is taken of how the research will be carried out. If it is trivial research, few concessions should be made to allow it to happen; if essential, then other moral imperatives may or may not be overruled. I discuss this balancing of different moral claims in much more detail when I come to consider duty- and right-based considerations. It is also the case that establishing the importance of the research goal matters in and of itself from a goal-based perspective, for the straightforward reason that an agent should not commence an action without first considering the morality of its consequences.

Researcher's motive a guide: problems with paying researchers to conduct research

Where the goal of a research proposal is not obviously related to immediate improvements in healthcare it could be argued that the guide to its acceptability lies in the motives of the researcher. He may wish to conduct his research from genuine scientific curiosity, or he may have a strong sense that a particular avenue of investigation will ultimately lead to real developments in his field of medicine, or he may have an overriding concern with the welfare of the patients in his discipline and want to help, albeit in a small way, to improve their lot. All these motives could be said to be pure.

Suppose, however, that he is being paid to conduct the research? Traditionally, research ethics committees have been suspicious of payments going into researchers' pockets (as distinct, say, from departmental funds). Pharmaceutical company fees for routine clinical research of drugs in development will often be paid directly to the researcher. Sometimes these fees are high. They are said to cover the researcher's time and expenses for running the trial. These costs are often considerable, and it is important that funds for ordinary treatments do not get diverted into pharmaceutical company research. But in the context of trying to decide what is important or necessary research, and relying to some extent on the researcher's motive as a guide for this decision, the fact that he is being paid inevitably raises a question about how important the research really is. (There are also questions about the justice of the researcher being paid when the research subjects are not. In the UK, for example, research subjects are only paid if the research is non-therapeutic. Payment to research subjects is discussed in Chapter Eight.)

Even if research funds are not going to individuals, or are not from commercial sources, there are still factors which can interfere with the researcher's motives for doing research. When research funds are applied for, the applicant will tailor his research proposal to fit the wishes of the grant-giving body, in order to secure the grant. Hence, the researcher is not as free as we might hope to act only for the best and purest motives. He has to do the best he can in the circumstances, and those who judge him need to recognize that.

Why researchers should always aim for the sky

The best treatment for any condition is the one that cures it completely and does so with no harmful side effects, either to the individual patient or to the wider environment. Every researcher probably has such a grand hope lurking somewhere at the back of his mind as he embarks on the long and laborious process of designing, carrying out and disseminating his research programme. It is a good hope to sustain and work towards, because it avoids the tacit assumption that medicine and other treatments must of necessity do harm, if good is also to be enjoyed. It might seem odd, to a lay person at any rate, that such a notion exists, but it does. It has been argued that that which could do no harm cannot, therefore and for that reason, effect a cure either. A researcher would not want to claim total success while further improvements are still possible. Hence, the research should always aim at absolute good, not because it will always achieve it, but because it is likely to get closer to it than if a less absolute goal is sought. If we aim at the centre of a target our arrows are more likely to hit it than if we only aim at the target.

Methods of research

Once a research goal has been identified we then have to work out how to achieve it in a reliable way. Different research questions require different research designs to answer them, if they are to be answered in a way that is widely recognized and accepted. This is a matter of good science, but it is also a matter of ethics, because research which is improperly designed is both a waste of resources and a source of potential harm if its conclusions are wrong and they are believed to be right. The choice of research method requires technical knowledge. There is room here to describe only briefly the basic principles of different research methods. I hope, however, to convey a sense of how each method tries to answer questions, in order to show why different questions need different ways of answering them. The three major types of research methods are: randomized controlled trials; observational research; and qualitative research. Some methods provide more objective means of measuring outcomes; others are more subjective.

Randomized controlled trials

The randomized controlled trial is the most well-recognized method of arriving at an objective answer to some sorts of research question. People often wrongly assign causes to events because what they think they see is not what is actually happening. The fact that a doctor gives a treatment to a person with condition X, and condition X goes away after she has had the treatment, does not mean that the treatment cures condition X. What the doctor saw in that case may be due to the treatment really working, or it may be due to a different cause, such as the condition of the patient, faulty measurements of the outcome, or chance. The randomized controlled trial seeks to avoid wrongly attributing treatment success to the medicine being tested, by factoring out anything that might give the wrong impression of the medicine. The most robustly designed controlled trial is the one which has factored out most causes of wrong attribution. This includes both patients' and doctors' attitudes towards and beliefs about the efficacy of a treatment.

The fundamental property of a controlled trial is that it makes a comparison, so that one group of patients receiving a new treatment will be compared to another group being given an existing, often standard treatment, a placebo (dummy treatment) or no treatment at all. The patients receiving the standard treatment, the placebo or no treatment are known as the control group, while those receiving the new treatment are the experimental group. Sometimes the groups change over after a defined period, so that the control group of patients become the experimental group and vice versa (crossover trial design). Sometimes the trial compares different doses of the same medicine. If possible, the treatments are masked, so that neither the patient nor the doctor knows which treatment the patient is receiving.

Patients will be randomly allocated to either of the two groups; no-one chooses who goes into which group. Randomization is effected by a method equivalent to tossing a coin, usually by computer. There are eligibility criteria for joining trials, not only for the safety of the patients, but also for ensuring that the groups are appropriate. Bias in the group membership can give rise to an apparent difference between the two treatments which would then be wrongly attributed to the treatment.

Assessment or measurement bias is avoided by ensuring that the measurements of results are objective, for example the patients' serum cholesterol or haemoglobin being tested by a machine in a laboratory. If, on the other hand, the assessment has to be based upon the clinician's judgement of the success of a treatment, or on the patients' self-report, then the assessments themselves are masked. This is achieved by ensuring either that the clinician doing the judging is not the clinician who administered the treatments, or, if it is patient self-report, the clinician assessing the reports does not know which patient said what.

To control the chances of errors in assigning causes, the sample size of research subjects must be sufficiently large, and the study must have an acceptable *p value* and adequate *power*. The *p* value is 'the probability that a difference at least as large as that seen in the data would occur by chance, if the true difference between the treatments is zero' (MacRae, 1996). Claiming a treatment difference when there is none is called a Type One, or Alpha, error. Conventionally, the hypothesis that the difference between the treatments is zero is rejected if the *p* value is lower than 5%. When the *p* value is lower than 5% the difference is referred to as being statistically significant.

The *power* of a study is its probability of not missing a real difference between the treatments. This is known as a Type Two, or Beta, error. The power of the study needs to be high, traditionally 80% or above. A power of 80% means that there is an 80% chance that the study will produce a statistically significant difference if the treatments are different from each other.

MacRae notes that whilst the calculation of the *p* value and the statistical power of the study requires mathematical expertise, the clinically relevant difference between the two treatments being compared, that is, the goal of the research, is a matter of value judgement and it is this which will determine the sample size needed. The greater the difference looked for between two treatments, the fewer the number of patients that are needed in the sample size. The way that the question is approached is to state the null hypothesis ('the true difference between the two treatments is zero') and then try to disprove it, which is much more scientifically sound than devising a positive hypothesis and trying to prove it (Popper, 1959).

Observational or epidemiological research

Most observational or epidemiological research involves observing what is happening without interfering, unlike experimental research, such as the controlled trial which intervenes and measures the effect of the intervention. Examples of exceptions to the rule of not interfering are studies of the effects of placing fluoride in the water supply to one area, or studying the effect of screening programmes for cancer in one area, where the fluoridization or the screening programme take place in order to be studied. Observational research can be either descriptive or analytic. Descriptive studies only describe phenomena without trying to identify cause and effect. Some descriptive studies are qualitative (see below), whilst others are quantitative, such as the large-scale surveys conducted by government agencies to measure the attitudes and habits of the population. Analytic studies do seek connections between cause and effect, namely, exposure and outcome, and they are always quantitative. There are three types of analytic observational research methods:

(a) **Cohort studies** compare two groups, one of which is exposed to a risk and one of which is not, and follow the two groups prospectively, calculating the ratio of rates of disease. Importantly, each group has chosen the exposure or lack of it (for example, smoking).
(b) **Case-control studies** start with the outcome and measure prior exposure. In effect, they seek to reconstruct a cohort study after the event, for example to discover the causes of rare disease events.
(c) **Cross-sectional studies** collect data on individuals at one point in time, for example the effect on people of a large-scale disaster. These studies cannot inform the researcher whether the observed effects came before or after the exposure, so they are not very reliable. (Thorogood, 1996)

Qualitative research

Qualitative research takes an interpretative approach to subject matter, studying things in their natural settings and attempting to make sense of or interpret phenomena in terms of the meanings that people bring to them. Qualitative research recognizes that there are many different ways of making sense of the world, and it is, therefore, concerned with discovering the meanings seen by the researched, rather than imposing the interpretation of the researchers (Jones, 1995). Because of this concern not to impose interpretative criteria on phenomena, the research methods are numerous and some are very loose indeed. A few of the different methods used by qualitative researchers are given here.

(a) **Observational methods** involve the researcher systematically watching people and events to find out about behaviours and interactions in normal settings (Mays and Pope, 1995).

(b) **Qualitative interviews** take many forms. There are three basic types: the structured interview, with a structured questionnaire; the semi-structured interview, with open-ended questions; and the in-depth interview, involving one or two issues covered in great detail, with the questions based on what the interviewee says (Britten, 1995).

(c) **Consensus methods** provide another means of synthesizing information than systematic review (see below), using a wider range of information and harnessing the insights of appropriate experts to enable decisions to be made. One commonly used consensus method is the Delphi process. This proceeds in a series of rounds, in which a series of expert opinions is generated and scored by experts until a consensus is reached. The other commonly used method is the nominal group technique, otherwise known as the expert panel (Jones and Hunter, 1995).

(d) **Focus groups** are a form of group interview that uses the communication between the members of the group to generate research data. Hence, group interaction is specifically part of the method. The method is useful for exploring people's knowledge and experience, and for examining not only what people think but why and how (Kitzinger, 1995).

(e) **Case study evaluation** involves studying the implementation of a policy or other intervention empirically, by evaluating case studies of the implementation. Qualitative or quantitative methods may be used. The tradition of using case studies in medicine is a long one; this is an attempt to systematize and extend that use (Keen and Packwood, 1995).

When to use which method

For a long time there have been fundamental differences of opinion about which research methods are reliable and valid for the discovery of knowledge which can then be believed by others. The randomized controlled trial, because of its ability to measure objectively, has taken top place in the hierarchy of evidence, and has provided the gold standard against which other research methods are measured. Hence, the less able a study is to prove something objectively, the less reliable and useful it is. We can consider how valid this claim is when we look at disseminating the results of research. However, I would point out here that to neglect other research methods is inappropriate, since some aspects of medicine are not amenable to randomized controlled trials. For example, if we wanted to know what the physically harmful effects of smoking were, we could not ethically answer that question by a randomized controlled trial, because it would involve random-ly allocating a group of people to smoke, which we know is bad for them. Or, if we wanted to know about patients' perceptions of a treatment we had administered to them, a randomized controlled trial would not tell us, because there is no prior hypothesis to determine the comparative groups to which patients should be allocated.

The following comments are helpful in showing the usefulness of the different research methods:

Randomized controlled trials carried out in specialised units by expert care givers, designed to determine whether an intervention does more good than harm under ideal conditions, cannot tell us how experimental treatments will fare in general use, nor can they identify rare side-effects. Non-experimental epidemiology can fill that gap. Similarly, because the theoretical concerns about the confounding of treatment with prognosis have been repeatedly confirmed in empirical studies..., non-experi-mental epidemiology cannot reliably distinguish false positive from true positive conclusions about efficacy. Randomized trials minimize the possibility of such error. And neither randomized trials nor non-experimental epidemiology are the best source of data on individuals' values and experiences in health care; qualitative research is essential. (Sackett and Wennberg, 1997)

Disseminating the results of research

Suppose that a researcher has found an ethical goal for his research, and designed and executed the research in a scientifically valid manner. He still needs to think about how to tell others about his results, and persuade them to alter their clinical practice on the basis of what he have discovered that is new. The difficulties that stand in his way arise from the unwillingness of individuals to change, from publication bias and from bad indexing. There is, in addition, a more fundamental question, which resonates with the dis-cussion in Chapter One. Is evidence-based medicine, that is, medicine which uses evidence from research, the best kind of medicine there is? Evidence-based medicine has a significant advantage over medicine practised solely according to hunches and subjective interpretations of past experience, but there are questions to be asked both about the underlying premise and about the practical utility of evidence-based medicine.

The following paragraphs will consider: the challenge of encouraging clinicians to put knowledge into practice; the challenge of bringing together all the information available from research; and questions about the basic idea of evidence-based medicine.

Encouraging clinicians to put knowledge into practice

There are numerous reasons for the difficulty of persuading clinicians to put the results of research into practice (*Lancet*, 1993). It may be that results are viewed with caution, with a desire to wait and see what happens when others try using them. Many doctors will have had the experience of hearing about promising new agents, backed by scientific studies, which have in the end been found wanting. There may be a fear of potential adverse side effects not yet shown in the research, or confusion over indications and contra-indications. A clinician may have had a previous bad experience with the treatment in question which overrides, in his mind, the less tangible benefits shown by the research. Cost effectiveness and quality of life evaluations in specific areas may make the application of the new treatment difficult to use by an individual doctor. This may be true if, for example, the new treatment requires more knowledge or skill, and more equipment or personnel. The clinician may simply not believe the research findings, either because he does not share the assumptive basis of the researcher, or because he thinks the measurements in the research are not rigorous enough.

The *Lancet* suggests ways in which doctors might be encouraged to put advances in medical knowledge into practice. The primary way it suggests is through education in journals and at postgraduate educational and scientific meetings. However, a cautionary tale is offered by researchers who conducted a randomized controlled trial of educational visits to enhance the use of systematic reviews in 25 obstetric units (Wyatt et al., 1998). They found that their visits made little difference to the practice in these units.

The *Lancet* also suggests that meta-analyses are useful because the cumulative evidence can be conveyed more quickly to a busy clinician. Doctors who are well-acquainted with the pathophysiology and natural history of a particular disorder are also more likely to put advances in knowledge into practice. If the doctor has actually participated as an investigator in research he will be more persuaded of a treatment's efficacy, having seen it for himself. The lesson from this, the *Lancet* states, is that trials need to be planned with the implementation of their results as part of the project.

Collecting the results of research

In 1991 Philippa Easterbrook and others discovered considerable publication bias in clinical research (Easterbrook et al., 1991). Their survey found that studies showing a statistically significant difference between the groups of patients receiving different treatments were more likely to be published than those finding no difference. Studies with significant results were also likely to lead to a greater number of publications and presentations, and to be published in journals with a high citation impact factor (likelihood of being quoted elsewhere). The bias was seen in all types of research, but especially in observational studies. This means that if a researcher had completed some research he would be far more likely to succeed in having it published if his results showed a difference between treatments. If his results were negative, that is, they showed that the experimental treatment was not, in fact, any different from its standard comparator, he would be less successful. The implication is that important negative results have not seen the light of day. Easterbrook concludes: 'These findings suggest that conclusions based only on a review of published data should be interpreted cautiously, especially for observational studies. Improved strategies are needed to identify the results of unpublished as well as published studies.'

In 1997 between 50 and 100 reputable medical journals called an amnesty for unpublished trials. Investigators with unreported trial data were invited to register their trials by completing an unreported trial registration form. The aim, said Roberts (1998), 'was to tap the silent subterranean pool of unpublished research and by bringing these data to the surface, to increase the power of systematic reviews and reduce the effects of publication bias'. At the time of writing, which was a year after the amnesty had been issued, Roberts reported that only 165 such trials had been registered. There was some involvement by the pharmaceutical industry, but government agencies on both sides of the Atlantic did not give their support, arguing that commercial confidentiality could not allow the pharmaceutical industry to tell all. Consequently, the amnesty was a flop.

Herxheimer had earlier anticipated that commercial and political secrecy would be an obstacle to the dissemination of research (Herxheimer, 1993). He stated that pharmaceutical companies, which might want to 'lose' results which did not demonstrate benefits of their treatments, as well as other sponsors of research, who might want to suppress results which were not politically desirable, thought that because they had funded and initiated the research they owned the results. This ignores the rights of research subjects, who participate because they think they are being useful to others. It also, argues Herxheimer, ignores the rights of investigators, who take overall moral responsibility for the proper conduct of their research, and the rights of the institutions where they do their work, which support them.

Another problem with relying on published research is that if we were to go to an index to find the publications we want, we would miss an important source of knowledge: letters published in journals following the publication of research results (Bhopal and Tonks, 1994). The letters which follow original papers are essential for correcting scientific error and contributing to peer review. An example of their importance is the study of the Bristol Cancer Help Centre. The Bristol Cancer Help Centre, as its name implies, offers treatment to people with cancer. Its methods involve no conventional or allopathic medicine; only a strict diet and much support at the spiritual and psychological level. The published study concluded that the Centre's treatments did not work. But there were a number of faults in the design of the research, which numerous subsequent letters pointed out. One of the letters was from the funding agency which withdrew its support from the main conclusions of the research. Gaining a proper sense of the results of the research would entail reading the letters as well as the original paper. Similarly, a paper published in the *British Medical Journal* in 1992 suggested that elective delivery by caesarean section of the breech fetus at term was far safer than spontaneous vaginal delivery. Nineteen letters robustly challenged the paper's conclusions; subsequent articles cited the paper, not the comments (Bhopal and Tonks, 1994). Internet indexing has improved this record.

Nevertheless, systematic reviews, as their name implies, are genuine attempts to review research evidence 'which has taken steps to avoid bias and the play of chance' (Chalmers, personal communication, 2000). Despite the challenges to the success of such projects, their contribution to the development of sound medical practice should be celebrated and supported.

The limitations of evidence-based medicine

Kerridge has evaluated the ideas underlying evidence-based medicine in a thoughtful article (Kerridge et al., 1998), and his observations on evidence-based medicine are resonant both of goal-based morality and of research in general. Kerridge agrees that evidence-based medicine is founded on a strong ethical and clinical ideal: it allows the best evaluated methods of healthcare to be identified and helps doctors and patients make more informed decisions. However, it is also an expression of consequentialism, which argues that an action can be assessed by measuring its consequences. Many important outcomes cannot be defined or measured. Whose interests should be taken into account when determining outcomes? Should systematic reviews include research projects which were conducted unethically? And what if the conclusions that a systematic review comes to are themselves intuitively morally abhorrent?

In medicine, says Kerridge, intangible values such as quality of life and justice are as important as quantifiable values such as mortality or cost. The systematic reviews and meta-analyses, on which evidence-based medicine relies, traditionally only recognize randomized controlled trials as substantial enough to merit a place in their review. This is understandable if the aim of systematic reviews is to provide objective knowledge, but this aim is inappropriate for medicine as a whole. Moreover, the problem of conclusions which are intuitively abhorrent is a real one. For example, a systematic review of treatments of the elderly may conclude that it is not economical to treat anyone over the age of 65. Arguably, however, no-one should be chary of discovering even unpalatable facts: the ethical questions arise over when and how to use them.

Using or not using the results of research which was conducted unethically presents problems in at least two respects for meta-analysis, and, indeed, for the amnesty called by editors of journals in 1997. It may be that a journal refused to publish a research paper because the way the research was conducted was unethical. This issue is discussed in Chapter Eight, citing a journal which faced exactly this dilemma of either turning down an article because the research it was based upon was unethical by 1990s standards, and losing the useful results of the work, or publishing it and giving a voice and platform to unethical practices, thereby encouraging them. Meta-analyses are only one step removed from the publications they use. Should the findings of unethical research be included in the reviews? Some answers to the question are looked at in Chapter Eight when the particular case is discussed.

In evidence-based medicine, randomized controlled trials are at the top of the hierarchy of reliable evidence. Controlled trials require the doctors to be happy for their patients to go into any of the different treatment groups for them to be able, ethically, to enrol their patients. Where the treatments being compared are roughly equivalent the doctor can do this. For interventions which have great benefits or which carry major risks, the doctor may well not be happy to allow his patients to be denied benefits or be exposed to risks. Colebrooke faced precisely this dilemma with penicillin in the 1930s (see Chapter Six). In such cases doctors may prefer to accrue evidence by reporting clinical observations or by using historical controls. For evidence-based medicine and the systematic reviews which support it, this relegates the evidence. The conflict between the need for scientifically reliable data and the need not to harm research participants is discussed again in Chapter Seven, in relation to placebo-controlled trials.

There are difficulties with using the evidence properly. Techniques for accurate application of trial results are needed. The crude application of results may, on average, do more good than harm, but they may none the less disadvantage some patients. If evidence is used as a basis for allocating funds, this will mean that only those treatments which have been tested by randomized controlled trials will be funded, and this means that only quantifiable treatments will be considered, or that treatments not amenable to being measured will none the less be subjected to inappropriate evaluations based on quantity rather than quality.

Kerridge implies that those who seek to practise evidence-based medicine are robotic and insensitive, which is unfair. Proponents of evidence-based medicine have to counter what they see as the real danger of doctors recommending treatments on the basis of experience and intuition when these can be so misleading. As I have said, I would not want to discount such practice, but I recognize the importance of balancing intuition with evidence, and hence the need for doctors to remain open to changing their practice. Whilst some research methods, mainly qualitative, try to measure systematically values other than quantifiable ones, in the hierarchy of evidence randomized controlled trials come top because they are capable of providing objective proof. Evidence-based medicine, then, relies most heavily on randomized controlled trials, and so do systematic reviews. This means that if anyone wants to use the results of research, and do so using systematic reviews, as the *Lancet* suggested, they will be relying mainly on quantifiable evidence, and many important aspects of medicine cannot be measured in this way.

It would be a mistake to be disheartened by the extensive list of difficulties with gathering and disseminating evidence. It is better to find out systematically whether a treatment works, even if it is difficult to persuade others of the validity of the work. And although evidence-based medicine should not be made into an absolute good, it is important for doctors to use evidence from research as well as their own experience and intuition when treating patients.

Summary and concluding remarks

If goal-based morality is used as part of the overall consideration of what makes a research project ethical, it has an important function, for it requires that the consequences of research projects be considered as matters of ethical concern. In other words, it brings what might be called the purely scientific considerations into the moral arena where, in my view, they certainly belong. The scientific questions relate to the goals of the research, the way the research is designed, and the dissemination of its results. Hence, a researcher needs to consider these issues in a morally responsible way. The most difficult issue is that of the goal of research. It is perfectly possible to give a scientific justification for conducting a research project in terms of its immediate goals of finding out, for example, whether a particular drug does in fact treat a particular symptom, or whether it is possible to grow human tissue from the stem cells of cloned embryos. It is more difficult to judge whether such questions should be asked in the first place. My own suggestions were that a researcher should consider the effects of his research at every level where it can have an effect, and that he should aim the research at the goal of finding treatments which are harmless to all.

Once a researcher has decided on the acceptability of a research project's goal, he then has to consider which of many research methods is the best to answer his research question. Different research questions require different research designs. Finally, he needs to disseminate the results. This too is a practical matter necessary for ethical reasons. Not to publish results takes away the overall goal-based justification for the research, which is for the greater good. Nevertheless, there are some real problems with dissemination and with the way results are used.

Once we have addressed these ethical considerations as best we can, the second third of the ethics of research on humans has to be addressed. This is related to what the research subjects will have to undergo for the research to take place. This ethical concern arises within the context of duty-based thinking, which is the subject of the next chapter.

3

Duty-based morality: acting in the research subjects' best interests

The foundations of duty-based thinking

From goals to duties

Utilitarianism asks no more of us as moral agents than that we consider the outcome of our actions. Provided that its outcome maximizes happiness, an action is morally justified. We are not asked to give an account of the rightness of the action itself. There are no principles to refer to for that sort of judgement. The last chapter found that the goals of research are important issues morally, but it is not enough to identify a good goal for research and leave the moral consideration at that, even if the related issues of scientific method and the dissemination of results are satisfactorily included. The conduct of the research itself has to be subjected to moral constraints. The example quoted from the Nuremberg Trials helped to show why. If someone's focus as a researcher is only on the outcome of her research, she is going to miss the ethical implications of what she has to do to arrive at that result. Goal-based morality cannot help us think about the ethics of the research procedures, because its focus is always on the future. We need a duty-based deontological moral approach rather than a teleological one to assist our analysis at this stage.

Duty-based deontological morality concerns itself specifically with the contents of an action rather than with its results. It considers actions in the light of explicit moral principles, which have to be identified and adhered to. In the context of research, some research which is aimed at highly desirable outcomes, involving significant steps forward in medical knowledge, may nevertheless be wrong according to a duty-based deontological approach because of what the research involves. For example, an experiment may necessitate harm to its subjects in order to gain scientifically sound results. The utilitarian may ask why the harm to a few should weigh sufficiently in the balance to prevent research whose goals will be significantly useful. The duty-based moralist needs to be able to say why it should, if indeed it should. In short, duty-based deontological morality should be able to give some substance to the intuitive notion that some actions are, like the Nazi doctors' experimentation, 'simply wrong'. This chapter will consider the strengths and weaknesses of the approach, and then see how to use it as part of a moral analysis of research on humans. Two formulations of duty-based ethics will be described and their practical use for our purposes will be investigated. The first formulation to be considered is the tradition of natural law ethics. The second is that of Immanuel Kant (1724–1804), who proposed an imperative moral law which was categorical, hence obligatory.

Natural law ethics

The moral principles of natural law ethics are derived from observable facts about nature. The best way to explain how this works is to give an example. In his treatise on fornication and marriage, Thomas Aquinas (1225/6–1274) derived a comprehensive package of moral teaching on the subject using arguments from natural law. One of his derived moral rules is that the marriage between a man and a woman should be for life. This is how he argues the point:

Besides, there is in men a certain natural solicitude to know their offspring. This is necessary for this reason: the child requires the father's direction for a long time. So, whenever there are obstacles to the ascertaining of offspring they are opposed to the natural instinct of the human species. But, if a husband could put away his wife, or a wife her husband, and have sexual relations with another person, certitude as to offspring would be precluded, for the wife would be united first with one man and later with another. So, it is contrary to the natural instinct of the human species for a wife to be separated from her husband. And thus, the union of male and female in the human species must be not only lasting, but also unbroken. (Aquinas, c. 1264 p. 147)

By identifying a 'natural' desire in a man to know his offspring, Aquinas finds a basis for the moral rule that a man and a woman should stay together for life. Where, however, does Aquinas derive his natural laws from? If they come from simple, empirical observation, his laws could be contested on their own grounds. For we could observe that a number of men do not, in fact, stay with their offspring, providing evidence of a lack of interest in them. If Aquinas gains his 'laws of nature' from his perception of what happens anyway, for every perception he had from which he derived a moral rule, one could think of a counter perception to undermine it. For his laws of nature, if they are to give rise to rules which we are supposed to obey (and can, therefore, choose *not* to obey), must be breakable. If he only identified laws of nature which we could not dispute, such as the law of gravity, he would have no need to devise a moral law from it, since the law of gravity is unbreakable. 'You must fall through the air at great speed if you jump out of a window' is not a moral law, it is a statement of fact, and the word 'must' means 'will', not 'ought to'.

We might rejoin, however, that although the law of gravity is unbreakable, it is possible to act as if it was. That is to say, you could decide to jump out of a window. The law of gravity does not remove your ability to do that. What it does do is to ensure that if you do 'break' the law, you will suffer the consequences. But for a short time, say while you were sitting on the window sill just before jumping, you might think that, in fact, you will not fall to the ground but will fly. Suppose that the desire of a man to know his offspring is equivalent to the law of gravity, and that his decision to leave his children is equivalent to jumping out of a window. He might not experience the consequences of his action to begin with, but he (and his children) might suffer later, just as the person falling to the ground will suffer after a (short) period has elapsed.

On this basis, we should be able to derive moral laws from observable facts of nature. We would need to find laws which are as unquestionable as the law of gravity, and then draw up rules which are the equivalent of telling people not to jump out of windows. It is worth noting that the reason for obeying these kinds of moral laws would be prudential rather than virtuous. It would not be in our interests to disobey them, if the consequences of doing so were the equivalent of hitting the ground after falling from a great height. In fact, it could be argued that these sorts of rules are not really moral at all. For although it is unintelligent to jump out of a window, it could hardly be called immoral to do so, or positively moral to refrain. Aquinas observed that the proper function of semen is to effect procreation, and for that reason it should not be used for any other purpose, such as pleasure alone. No one would dispute that semen fertilizes eggs, but many people do not think it follows from that fact that it is immoral to have sexual intercourse using contraception. Would it be immoral to 'break' the law of gravity by flying an aeroplane?

What such a morality requires us to have is a belief that things have proper functions and it is right for us to ensure that those proper functions are fulfilled. If we want to know what is intrinsically right and wrong, we need to look at the function of the thing we are dealing with. If an action helps it fulfil its function, then the action is right. This sort of contention sounds trivial when it is applied to an eye, or a kidney, for although those things have definable functions it is hardly a matter of morality to ensure that they fulfil them. But in the context of medicine the approach becomes more meaning-ful. A doctor, by virtue of her professional title, has a particular role to play in relation to patients, that is, she owes them a duty of care, usually expressed as the duty to act in their best interests. This *is* her function, and it is uncontentious to assert that she *ought* to fulfil her function. She could choose not to, but this would be called wrong, again, uncontentiously. Moreover, the sense in which it is 'simply right' for a doctor to act in her patients' best interests is more akin to the law of gravity being 'simply right' than, say, not taking illegal drugs is 'simply right'. That drug-taking is wrong is subject to the circum-stances in which it happens. Smoking marijuana in order to heighten sensory experiences might be wrong. Smoking it to alleviate the symptoms of multiple sclerosis might not be. At least the different circumstances merit a discussion. The law of gravity cannot be contested in the same way, and neither can the doctor's duty to act in her patient's best interests. This is because the title 'doctor' defines the function which the person who takes that title has to perform. If she did not want to act in her patients' best interests, she would not call herself a doctor. Now, if she also wishes to conduct research upon her patients, and hence add the title 'researcher' to the title doctor, a question arises as to whether it can still be taken as read that she must act in her patients' best interests. I would argue that such a function remains so long as the title doctor remains, which it will do if there is someone present calling himself a patient. It is even questionable whether doctors can shed their role at any time (Walsh, 1998). The role of researcher has its functions and associated duties, and a case would need to be made for the doctor's duty to care to override the researcher's duty to extend medical knowledge. The case can be made by considering the situation if the researcher's role was allowed to override that of the doctor. This would mean that in a research project, were a participant to show signs of distress, but his coming out of the trial would jeopardize the trial, the doctor/researcher ought to keep him in the trial. On the contrary, the first consideration should be the well-being of the patient/participant, and the doctor's duty to care takes precedence.

Kant's categorical imperative

A different, though related, basis for duty-based deontological morality can be found in the philosophy of Immanuel Kant. Kant argued that pure reason, by its very existence, warranted moral behaviour. Human beings, having this faculty of reason, are therefore bound by the moral law. His argument, as described in his *Fundamental Principles of the Metaphysic of Morals* (1785), develops as follows:

Reason, given to rational beings by Nature, is capable of recognizing absolute truth, stripped of all empirical qualifications. Reason is, therefore, autonomous, needing no external assistance to help it recognize what is true. Reason directs the will, which, if obedient, overrides personal inclinations. The will, properly directed, expresses itself as the motive of duty. Actions which have moral worth are those which are performed solely from the motive of duty and not for any other reason whatsoever. The motive of duty is determined by the maxim or law according to which the action is performed, which our reason recognizes and accepts. The absolute maxim or law which governs our actions is called the *categorical imperative*.

The categorical imperative, if it is to be shown to be absolutely required, will not have its truth demonstrated by experience or by reference to the empirical world. Indeed, we will not be able to say that we have ever seen an act which has moral worth, because we will not know if personal inclination had any part in its motivation. The example of others, reference to God, or any other medley of external justifications or inspirations for moral behaviour, cannot provide the basis for our actions, for such justifications are subject to change and are therefore unreliable. The categorical imperative has to be demonstrated conceptually in order to be recognized by our autonomous reason. Kant identifies the following categorical imperatives: (i) act in such a way that the maxim governing your action *can be* a universal law of nature; and (ii) act in such a way *that you can at the same time will* that the maxim governing your action can be a universal law of nature. These, Kant argues, are moral laws which apply in all circumstances and are absolutely required of reason. It may be that in practice we do not follow the categorical imperative, but this is not because it is not absolutely required of us as rational beings. We fail to follow it because our inclinations are at odds with our reason, and our will, which could override our inclinations, is not obedient to our reason.

Kant offers some examples of the application of the categorical imperative. Here is one of them:

A man reduced to despair by a series of misfortunes feels wearied of life, but is still so far in possession of his reason that he can ask himself whether it would not be contrary to his duty to himself to take his own life. Now he inquires whether the maxim of his action could become a universal law of nature. His maxim is: From self-love I adopt it as a principle to shorten my life when its longer duration is likely to bring more evil than satisfaction. It is asked then simply whether this principle founded on self-love can become a universal law of nature. Now we see at once that a system of nature of which it should be a law to destroy life by means of the very feeling whose special nature it is to impel to the improvement of life would contradict itself, and therefore could not exist as a system of nature; hence that maxim cannot possibly exist as a universal law of nature, and consequently would be wholly inconsistent with the supreme principle of duty. (Kant, 1785, p. 50)

The maxim has to be capable of being universalized, but it also has to be consistent for the moral agent to will it to be universalized. Here is another example:

A ... [man], who is in prosperity, while he sees that others have to contend with great wretchedness and that he could help them, thinks: What concern is it of mine? Let everyone be as happy as heaven pleases, or as he can make himself; I will take nothing from him nor even envy him, only I do not wish to contribute anything to his welfare or his assistance in distress! Now no doubt if such a mode of thinking were a universal law, the human race might very well subsist, and doubtless even better than in a state in which everyone talks of sympathy and good-will, or even takes care occasionally to put it into practice, but on the other side, also cheats when he can, betrays the rights of men, or otherwise violates them. But although it is possible that a universal law of nature might exist in accordance with that maxim, it is impossible to *will* that such a principle should have the universal validity of a law of nature. For a will which resolved this would contradict itself, inasmuch as many cases might occur in which one would have need of the love and sympathy of others, and in which, by such a law of nature, sprung from his own will, he would deprive himself of all hope of the aid he desires. (Kant, 1785 p. 51–2)

Notice that Kant is concerned, not to persuade us that such actions are wrong for consequentialist reasons, or that they are undesirable, but rather that they are inconsistent. The categorical imperative does not ask, as rule utilitarianism might ask, How would we like to live in a world where people did not help each other? Rather it is asking whether it is logically possible for the person who wants 'not to help others' to will that that principle be followed universally. Hence, for a rational being whose nature is to behave reasonably, such actions are categorically forbidden. There can be no argument as to their being wrong, for they go against the tenets of reason. It is rather like the absolute requirement on a doctor to act in her patients' best interests because she is a doctor and for no other, external purpose. She does not do it because it is a good thing to do, but because it is rational, if she calls herself a doctor, to behave like one. In the same way, reason, by its own nature, accepts the validity of the categorical imperative, because the categorical imperative is rational. By virtue of being reasonable, we are obliged to obey it. We could ignore it, but if we do so, then we can no longer claim to be reasonable people. Following reason, or acting like a doctor if that person is one, has good consequences because it makes us behave well, but we do not do it because it is good, or because we feel altruistic, or because of some intuitive idea of what is right, but because it is right in the same way that the law of gravity is right. Here, then, is our robust deontological moral principle to withstand the force of consequentialist arguments if we need to.

Duty-based moral thinking applied to medical research

The two examples of duty-based deontological ethics examined so far have yielded some useful fruit. Natural law ethics suffers from the difficulty of establishing facts of nature. However, it helps a doctor identify where her duty lies. It can be postulated that, as a doctor, someone's 'natural' function is to act in the best interests of her patients, and that it is as much her natural function to do that as it is for bodies to fall through the air. Kant postulated that reason, by its autonomous nature, is bound by the categorical imperative absolutely, because the categorical imperative is reasonable in and of itself, without any need for external justification. By her nature as a rational being, then, a doctor has no need to add a further justification for acting in this way according to the categorical imperative. Just as a rational being will naturally act according to reason, so a doctor will naturally owe a duty of care to her patients.

From this 'natural law' that a doctor must always act in her patients' best interests, we can derive a duty-based approach to medical research on humans, in all cases where research is conducted by a doctor, or other healthcare professional whose relationship with patients has similar priority over other duties. Although the function of researcher has its own set of important duties, these do not override those of the doctor's function and must necessarily give way should the need arise.

Although the duty to care of a doctor overrides the duty to do good-quality research of a researcher, it need not follow that absolutely any risk of harm to the patient/participant has to be removed before his doctor can rightly ask him to take part in research. It might in any case be a strong wish of the patient that he participate in a trial that exposes him to some risk but is of great potential benefit to future patients. Such a wish need not be ignored, but the doctor's duty to care entails that any risk should be minimized. A view must be taken as to what constitutes too great a risk to ask a patient to face. In coming to such a view, the doctor should not let the researcher's zeal for results overcome her primary concern for her patient's well-being. It is a matter of striking a balance, but the decision should err on the side of the patient's interests, not those of science and society (World Medical Association, 1996).

In order to take a duty-based approach to the ethics of research we need to know what the research is going to involve for the research participants. This means that we need to complete the goal-based analysis first, for that will tell us what the research method is and, therefore, what procedures the participants will have to undergo. For example, a randomized controlled trial will involve the blind allocation of different treatments to patients. Outcome measures like urine analysis or blood sugar levels will involve peeing in a bottle or extra needles, and so on.

As I found in the earlier discussion, the duty-based principle which will govern the analysis of a research project's procedures is derived from the doctor's duty to care for her patient, that is, to act in his best interests. As I suggested, this duty is absolute, not contingent upon other factors being in place. The doctor's duty to care expresses itself in offering to her patient those treatments which are in his best interests, and avoiding doing anything to him that is harmful. If, by virtue of being in a research project, he will be exposed either to treatments which are of no benefit, or to actions which may cause him harm, then it is duty-based morality which will call the ethical acceptability of the research into question. Goal-based morality will be concerned with the potential good towards which the research is aiming. Right-based morality will want to know if the participant is willing to be harmed, and will not consider that it may be inappropriate to ask him in the first place. Hence duty-based morality plays an essential part in the analysis of the ethics of research on humans.

It was said earlier that the duty-based principle to be applied to research on humans is that of benefiting and not harming the research participants. Applying the principle involves subjecting research procedures to scrutiny against this yardstick. It is helpful, in doing this, to separate research into therapeutic and non-therapeutic types, because different levels of benefit and harm can be expected and justified in each. Therapeutic research is research which is conducted in the context of clinical care: the participants in the research project are patients expecting to be treated for their illness as well as to help the researcher gain knowledge which can be generalized. In this context some harm to the research subject might be expected, but it would be experienced as a necessary part of the therapy, and would be outweighed *in the individual research subject* by the therapeutic benefits he may enjoy from the treatment, be it experimental or standard. For example, treatment for cancer is associated with risks of some very unpleasant side effects, but the risks are outweighed by the therapeutic benefit, and the two are directly related. If a research project involved giving chemotherapy to a cancer sufferer, harm might be anticipated, but balancing benefit would also be anticipated, sufficient to render the harm acceptable.

By contrast, non-therapeutic research will offer no treatment to research participants; they are simply guinea pigs and can expect no therapeutic benefit from being in the research project. Strictly speaking, duty-based morality demands that participants of non-therapeutic research be exposed to no risk of harm, since there is no balancing benefit to them. Weighing risk of harm to individual research participants against benefit to future other people is the function of goal-based moral thinking, not that of duty-based thinking. But it is impossible to remove absolutely all risk of harm from non-therapeutic research.

The key to determining whether any given research project is therapeutic or non-therapeutic is to look at the intention of the researcher. If she wishes only to generate new knowledge then the research is non-therapeutic. If, however, she wishes to treat the patient in front of her as well as gain further knowledge from treating him, then the research is therapeutic. Typically, therapeutic research involves randomized controlled trials, in which treatments are allocated to groups of patients in a blinded fashion, so as to discover, with as little bias as possible, which of the treatments being compared is better. Non-therapeutic research can take many forms, from studies of drugs being administered for the first time to healthy humans, to questionnaire surveys of large populations.

The application of duty-based thinking

Therapeutic research

Therapeutic research involves the intention to treat as well as the intention to gain knowledge which can be generalized. Hence, it will always take place in a medical setting, and the participants will be patients as well as experimental subjects. As was said earlier, therapeutic research usually takes the form of the randomized controlled trial. There are two ways in which randomized controlled trials can pose moral questions from a duty-based perspective. These are, first, that they may not offer patients in the trial the best treatment available, which it is the doctor's duty to provide; and second, there may be risks of harm which are not directly related to the therapeutic benefit anticipated from the treatments received in the trial. On the positive side, therapeutic research can offer benefits to patients in the form of more care and attention because of more resources available to the research team.

The reason a randomized controlled trial is set up is either because there is some doubt about a treatment which has hitherto been offered as a standard therapy or, more commonly, because a new treatment is being developed which is thought to be an improvement on any current treatment. The most objective and reliable way to show that one is better than another, or at least that one is not the same as another (Popper, 1959), is by gathering together a group of patients who have presented with the condition which needs treatment, and randomly allocating to each of them either the standard treatment or the experimental treatment. Importantly, the allocation of treatments is done not by preference of doctor or patient, but randomly, by the equivalent of tossing a coin. In this way, if a difference is seen in the outcome of treatment between the two groups of patients, it can be attributed to differences in the treatments the patients were given, and not, for example, because the patients, having chosen their treatment, feel more positive about it and display improvements for that reason. This research method is good for the goal-based purpose of answering the research question objectively. In this chapter we have to decide whether it is good by duty-based standards as well. Therefore, we will consider the design of randomized controlled trials from the point of view of discovering whether the doctor's duty to care first and foremost for her patient is able to be sustained in this specific context.

Definitions of equipoise

Equipoise is the name given to the attitude the doctor should have to the different treatments in a randomized controlled trial. By the nature of the trial design, the doctor will have no say in which of the treatment options in the trial her patients will receive. From a duty-based perspective, she will need to be entirely happy that such a situation is in her patients' best interests. This entails that she should have no preference for any of the treatments. She should genuinely believe that each treatment option in the trial is as good as any other. I shall call this attitude 'strong equipoise'.

Kennedy and others argue that such a balanced perspective is unlikely:

> A doctor may be involved in a trial which is designed to compare two treatments, both of which have their supporters. The doctor may have a preference for one form of treatment, although he has no evidence of a scientific nature to justify his preference. It may be based on experience, hunch, or some other reason; but whatever the reason, he has a preference. (Kennedy, 1988, p. 219)

However, many would argue that such an attitude is not ethically incompatible with becoming a researcher in a trial. Providing that the doctor remains uncertain that her preference is correct, she is still in equipoise. The doctor may have a preference, for after all she is unlikely to be proposing research into a new treatment if she does not think that, in the end, such a treatment will be better. I will call this form of equipoise 'weak equipoise'. Some will go further even than this, and, requiring no uncertainty from individual doctors, will merely require that there is uncertainty or differences of opinion across the relevant clinical community. Thus, individual doctors may strongly prefer one treatment over another, but as a group there are roughly equal divisions between them as to which is preferable. I shall call this 'community equipoise'.

From a goal-based perspective, both weak and community equipoise require research to be conducted on the treatments in question, so that the hunches and feelings of doctors can be tested objectively, and certainty achieved as to which treatment is better. From a duty-based perspective, however, it may be that only strong equipoise is sufficient for the doctor's duty to care to be honoured. Kennedy argues:

> Now, if it is accepted that the therapeutic relationship between doctor and patient is most successful when the doctor has faith in the treatment he is giving his patient, and this faith is reflected also in the trust which the patient has in the doctor, it will be clear that by adopting a form of treatment in which he has less confidence, the doctor may be aiding the pursuit of knowledge, but doing so by opting for a less than optimum relationship with his patient... If the doctor genuinely has no preference, then the problem does not arise, although I would submit that this is a comparatively rare occurrence. (Kennedy, 1988, p. 219)

Others would say that the duty to care is still maintained in weak and community equipoise because objectively there is equipoise, even if subjectively there is not. But it is also true to say that the objective equipoise is only there by virtue of (a collection of) subjective attitudes, some of which may be strongly held. It is the individual doctor who has to ask her patients if they want to participate in research, and it is, therefore, she as an individual who has to take responsibility for her decision whether or not to do so. Moreover, her patients will want to know what she really thinks and believes, and they are likely to be affected by her preferences. Arguably, then, only strong equipoise will do, and this, as has been indicated, is rare.

The different views given here about the extent to which the setting of a clinical trial is capable of allowing a doctor to act in her patients' best interests are crucial to the ethics of clinical research. If, by putting her patients into a clinical trial, a doctor is acting in their best interests, then the therapeutic research project should be considered in exactly the same way as ordinary therapy. In the ordinary therapeutic setting, certain rules apply which are not currently considered appropriate for research. For example, if a patient is unable to consent (incompetent) and needs treatment, it is legally up to his doctor to act in his best interests. If putting a patient into a clinical trial is the same as treating him in the ordinary way, and a clinical trial is currently underway involving patients with his condition, then that patient should be put into the clinical trial, regardless of the fact that he is unable to give his consent, for it is the doctor's duty to enrol him. If, on the other hand, it is not acting in her patients' best interests to enrol them in a trial, the incompetent patient will not automatically qualify.

I share Kennedy's view of the likelihood of a doctor having preferences, and the effect of such preferences on her patients. However, it may be objectively the case that a doctor's preference is based on bad evidence. The doctor may be part of a community in equipoise, that is, where there are differing views about which treatment is better. If she is positioned in this way, she ought in fact to notice the current thinking about the treatment for which she has a strong preference, educate herself out of her strong preference and join the strong equipoise group instead. In that way, both objectively and subjectively her duty to care is honoured if she then asks her patients to take part in a trial of the treatments.

Can patients still think their doctors are giving them individualized treatment if they are also participants in their trials?

Strong equipoise indicates that a doctor is convinced of her uncertainty about the comparative merits of different treatments. There is another aspect of the doctor's duty to care to which I referred in Chapter One, which is not really covered by the doctor being in strong equipoise. This is the matter of the patient receiving individualized care from his doctor. Even if the doctor is impartial as to the treatment choices, does the very act of enrolling her patient in a trial remove the possibility of her treating him as an individual in his own right, with specific medical needs and peculiarities? There are two ways in which a doctor can ensure that this loss of care does not occur. The first is that she should give consideration as to whether taking part in a trial is in his best interests, not just as regards the different treatments but also as regards his personal well-being. She should be able to establish this by asking him whether he would be happy to receive his treatment in the context of a trial. Second, the doctor should ensure that the research is designed in such a way that she or her research team can respond to particular medical needs as they arise. The result of the research should not depend upon having to ignore individual medical needs. Where needs cannot be anticipated or woven into the research design, it must be accepted that a patient can withdraw himself or be withdrawn from a trial should it be necessary.

Additional, non-therapeutic tests demanded by the research protocol

The second way in which therapeutic research can trouble duty-based morality is that participation in a clinical trial does not merely involve random allocation to a treatment that a patient might have had anyway or to a novel treatment. It also involves additional tests and measurements, such as urine or blood tests, in order to gain the results of the research. Hence, more is required of the patient in a trial than receiving treatment. It was suggested earlier that patients do better in clinical trials for precisely this reason: they receive far more attention, usually from more senior doctors, than they would if they were normal patients. The additional tests may, however, be irksome to patients as well as exposing them to further risks. Whichever is true, and it probably depends much upon the individual patient, these extra tests further emphasize the fact that being in a trial is not the same as receiving treatment in the ordinary way.

Where do these two problems with therapeutic research leave the ethical enquiry? From a duty-based perspective the focus has to return to the doctor who is conducting the research. The arguments about just how uncertain she has to be about the different treatments in the trial for her duty of care to remain intact are not objectively resolvable. It has, I submit, to remain a matter for each doctor's conscience and sense of duty to educate herself. For the duty-based requirement to be met, she must be satisfied that the patients whom she asks to enrol into the trial will receive as good a treatment as possible, whichever arm of the trial they are allocated to. It has to remain the doctor's decision for it is her duty to care which is at stake. Similarly, she must consider for whom of her patients the additional tests and measurements that come as part of the trial would be burdensome, and for whom they would not. Again, her duty will be to ensure that those for whom it would be disadvantageous should be excluded. The somewhat paternalistic ring to this suggestion will be considered below, when looking at non-therapeutic research.

The use of placebo

It is worth glancing briefly (this subject is considered in much more detail in Chapter Seven) at the use of placebo (pretend medicine, from the Latin *placere*, to please) in clinical trials, because it is a good example of where

goal-based and duty-based considerations can clash. The goal-based justification for a placebo arm in a trial is considerable. It adds scientific weight to the
design and its inclusion as one of the arms of the study often means that
smaller numbers need to be studied, and therefore fewer patients are required
to be research subjects. Hence, on utilitarian grounds, the use of placebos is
justified. However, the duty-based requirement to ensure that each individual in a trial is properly treated means that there is no justification for giving
some patients a worse treatment than others, simply in order for there to be
fewer subjects receiving the inferior treatment. The patient for whom the
doctor has a duty to care is the patient who is in front of her, not the
generality of patients. Placebo is only justified as part of a clinical trial if, as
described above, it can be offered by a doctor to her patient in the certainty
that this 'treatment' is at least as good as the other treatments. So, for
example, where there is no 'proven, available treatment' (World Medical
Association, 1996), a placebo arm is justified. Sometimes, confusingly, there
are treatments which have become standard without ever having had their
efficacy tested and hence are not 'proven'. New treatments could sometimes
justifiably be compared to these and to placebo as well. Each case would need
to be tested on its own merits. But from a duty-based perspective the moral
test is whether each patient in the trial is being treated in his best interests. It
is not to ensure scientific validity, nor to keep the patient numbers down.

Non-therapeutic research

Non-therapeutic research consists of research which has no therapeutic
aspect to it for the research participants. The researcher does not intend to
treat them: they are in the true sense her guinea pigs, unlike therapeutic
research participants, who are still also patients being treated. Examples of
non-therapeutic research include Phase I, 'first time in humans' studies to
measure toxicity and pharmacokinetics (where the drug goes and how long it
spends in the human body before being broken down or evacuated); research
into new forms of diagnosis; survey-type research, etc.

Does it matter that the best interests test fails in non-therapeutic research?

We could apply a strict interpretation of duty-based morality and argue that
non-therapeutic research is not morally acceptable under any circumstances,
because there is no therapeutic benefit, and there may be some risk. But why
should a person be prevented from being altruistic and exposing himself to
risks for the sake of others, if he wants to? There are plenty of risks which
people willingly take for no good moral reason (like recreational scuba
diving); this is taking a risk for a good reason: the benefit of others.

If we accept this argument about non-therapeutic research, however, we have to take a consistent line with the acceptability of the extra tests therapeutic research would entail, which are also, taken on their own, non-therapeutic. To put the decision of which of her patients would be burdened by the extra tests in the hands of the doctor, is paternalistic. Surely the better approach to the acceptability of non-therapeutic research, or the extra tests in therapeutic research, is to ask people if they are willing to expose themselves to risks, and only enrol them in the research if they are? Should duty-based morality stand aside for this right-based view, or should it hold its ground? The right-based view, which has intuitive merit, hangs upon the seeking and obtaining of consent. The next chapter will consider this aspect in detail. At this juncture, I shall find sufficient problems with relying on consent as the single moral determinant of whether research is too risky to support the argument that doctors should not cease to give careful consideration to what they ask people to consent to.

Should consent be the deciding factor?

The view that consent is what determines whether a non-therapeutic research project goes ahead may be put as follows: if a person is willing to become a research subject then he can be enrolled in the research, and if he is not, then he should be excluded. But this simple view is based upon a number of potentially false premises.

First, it relies on the belief that an action becomes right if a person wants it to happen. On its own this is not enough, just as it is not enough that a person should want someone to stab him to death to make the actual stabbing to death morally justified. That person's views on the matter may be significant, but they are not all that is needed in the moral consideration. Similarly, a research project does not become right just by virtue of the research participants wanting to be subjects.

Second, the view assumes that the elements of consent have been fulfilled, namely, that adequate information has been successfully imparted to a competent person whose subsequent agreement is voluntary. In particular, the voluntary nature of the decision may not be valid. If a doctor asks a patient to do something, or to take something, the patient's natural assumption will be that, if it does not benefit him, at least it will not harm him, since the function of doctors is to act in their patients' best interests. The trust that that is so is an essential part of the doctor–patient relationship. Once a patient starts to believe that a doctor might not have his interests at heart, he is simply not going to do what she says he needs to do in order to get better, particularly if the treatment is unpleasant. In fact, he may stop seeing her. He is likely, therefore, to agree, not because he has made an informed decision, but because his doctor has asked him.

Judgement of acceptability of risk remains with the researcher
To ask the participant to be the one who decides whether a risk in a non-therapeutic research project is too great to justify the research is, frankly, unfair. The onus remains on the doctor/researcher not to ask her patient to do something that is bad for him. The question of what makes risks in a non-therapeutic research project acceptable remains, then, with the researcher. It is up to her only to ask her participants to undergo procedures which are at an acceptable level of risk. Of course she must ask them before enrolling them into the research (and in that way give the opportunity to behave altruistically); that is not being questioned here. What is being questioned is the extent to which the doctor must play a part in shielding her patients from making risk assessments about factors that they should simply not be asked to consider. I would argue that the doctor must decide what risks are too great to be undertaken by the participants both in the therapeutic and the non-therapeutic context.

Summary and concluding remarks

This chapter has described two foundations of duty-based morality which give rise to the need to consider research from this perspective. These foundations were, first, that of natural law ethics, and second, the Kantian categorical imperatives, absolutely required of all rational beings. Natural law ethics provides principles of moral behaviour which are predicated on a belief that everything has a function which it is right for it to fulfil. Kant's categorical imperatives demand that we act in such a way that we can consistently will that the maxim governing our actions can become a universal law, and that the maxim is capable of becoming a universal law. Both these foundations point to a duty-based principle in the context of medicine, which is that the doctor has a duty to care for her patient. If the doctor is also a researcher, the doctor's duty to care overrides the researcher's duty to achieve reliable research results. The duty lies within the function of doctor. If a doctor's patients are to be used as research participants then they should be given the same level of care and consideration as they would be if they were patients in the ordinary way.

In therapeutic research the doctor has to be entirely happy to allow her patients to be randomly allocated to either or any of the treatments in a trial, including placebo, if there is a placebo arm, before she can rightly ask them to participate. This raises difficult questions about the degree of uncertainty she may have about the comparative efficacy of the different options.

In non-therapeutic research, the researcher must be satisfied that any risks to research participants are acceptable for each of the participants, not by being weighed against benefits to future patients.

The duty-based perspective on a research proposal provides a balancing set of moral concerns to those from the goal-based perspective. Duty-based concerns demand that research is conducted in such a way that research subjects are not harmed, or their exposure to harm is kept to a minimum in the case of non-therapeutic research, and that their best interests are served in therapeutic research. In this way, research subjects can be reassured that they will each be treated as separately important individuals to whom duties are owed, and not merely as instruments to a greater goal.

4

Right-based morality: respecting the autonomy of research participants

The foundations of right-based thinking

From duties to rights

The last chapter distilled from deontological ethical theories a duty-based approach to the ethics of research on humans, which stated that doctors owe a duty of care to their patients, and must therefore act in their best interests. This duty has traditionally bound doctors to behave ethically, but it has also created an ethos of paternalism in which the doctor has been thought to know best, gives orders, and is unassailably right in his decisions. Another kind of deontological ethics not yet discussed is based on people's rights. Rights can be a useful counterbalance to the duty-based moralist's tendency to be paternalistic.

Ian Kennedy argues: 'Historically, those who enjoy (in all senses of the term) power have insisted on the language of duty to express the relationship between the powerful and the rest' (1988, p. 391). People who are responsible for others have duties towards them. But although the language of duty can be invoked positively, as a way of determining how that responsibility will be carried out so that the good of all is served, it can also be used as a means of retaining power to the detriment of those purportedly being served. Just because a doctor believes he knows what is best for his patient, and just because he feels that he is doing his duty by his patient, it does not follow that what he proposes should happen. Kennedy would argue that unless some restraint, outside his own control, is put upon the doctor, abuse of his power can follow. Hence, some intrinsic powers need to be given to the weaker party, and these can be called her rights. Put in the context of medical research, this consists of only using a patient as a research subject if she wants to be so used, not because it is the doctor's self-appointed duty to consult his patient's wishes, but because the patient has an inherent right to self-determination.

Arguably the doctor's duty to consult and the patient's right to be consulted amount to the same thing. If the doctor's duty is sufficiently enforceable so that he has no choice but to consult his patient's wishes, what is the difference between that and asserting that the patient has a right to be consulted? The answer, replies Waldron (1995), is the basis upon which such a moral claim is made. If the reason we claim that a patient's wishes should be consulted is that it is her right, then we are asserting a right-based morality; if it is on the basis of the doctor's duty, then a duty-based morality. The reason the distinction is important is that the focus of moral thinking shifts between the agent of the action and the one most affected by it. If our morality is fundamentally duty-based, then the reason that we regard it as wrong to enter patients into research projects without their consent is that the researcher is violating his moral integrity by using people as a means to an end. If our morality is right-based, then it is the denial of the right of a patient to exercise her autonomy that is the fundamental problem. In the latter situation, it is not the moral health of the researcher we are concerned with, but the interests or rights of the research subject.

Immanuel Kant's theory of the autonomy of reason has often been invoked by right-based moralists to support the existence of inherent rights. Kant argues that rational beings should always be used as ends in themselves, and never merely as a means to another's end. But he argues this because it is incumbent upon rational beings to do their duty according to the precepts of reason, as said in the previous chapter. The duty of a rational being with regard to other rational beings is to treat them as ends in themselves. This is demanded by practical reason, and not by the construction or discovery of a right inherent in the one done unto. However, for Kant, it is precisely the prior existence of autonomous reason in a rational being that demands that we *should* treat her as an end in herself. This is an important observation for the way in which I am going to develop the use of right-based morality, so I shall return to Kant's moral theory later in the chapter.

If we are to assert that rights have a substantial existence which is capable of practical recognition, we have first to explain what is meant by someone having a right to something. We then have to show that that right is valid. Finally we have to show the practical application of the right-based approach in the context of medical research on human beings.

Definitions of rights

The Hohenfeldian cluster
If the statement: 'P has a right to X' is made, it can be meant in a number of different ways. For the following explanation I am grateful to Waldron for his summary of Hohenfeld's differentiation of meanings of rights (Waldron, 1995).
  (i) **P has no duty not to do X.** For example, an ambulance driver has the right to ignore road laws, by going through red traffic lights or driving on the wrong side of the road. Hohenfeld calls this kind of right a 'privilege'. This right, to avoid the criticism of being selfish, has to be

enjoyed only in the context of a particular service someone needs to perform. It has no merit if it is merely expressed in the childish assertion that whilst others may be bound by certain conventions and manners, I on the other hand am exempt, for no other reason than that I want to be. There can be no intrinsic reason for a person to hold the right which is a privilege: it must come with the function the person is called upon to perform. An ambulance driver who switched on his van's siren and broke road laws just because he was bored of waiting in traffic with the rest of the population, and not in order to fulfil his duty, would be abusing his privilege.

If this definition is turned around to state that P has no duty to do X, then it could be argued that patients have a right not to take part in research. Some, however, argue that no such right exists automatically, because patients now enjoy the fruits of previous patients' participation in research, and they have a duty to offer themselves as subjects in order to give back similar benefits to those they have received, for the sake of future patients.

(ii) **Everyone has a duty to let P do X.** This duty, which is contingent on the existence of certain rights, ranges from the negative duty not to impede P's action, to the positive duty to do what we can to make it possible for P to achieve X. These rights are called 'claim-rights'. Waldron notes that some of them are absolute, such as the right not to be imprisoned without due process, and some are contingent, such as the property rights over an item which has been purchased. The difficulty with this definition of a right lies in identifying what rights may be asserted in this way, and in whether someone has passive or active duties in respect of them. Even the passive duty of allowing us our freedom to act as we wish is questionable in some cases. If a child, for example, wishes to exercise her freedom in a way with which her parents are unhappy, do her parents have to accept that she is a free agent and they have a duty not to interfere, or does she *not* have that right? The age of the child will usually be the significant factor in this kind of decision. Another right that might be asserted is the right of a woman to have children. If she does have that right, is the contingent duty of everyone else simply not to prevent her from having a family, or is it our duty to take steps to ensure that she can have a family? We might have no difficulty in accepting that we owe other people the space and freedom to exercise their own wills over their own lives, if they want. But the woman who is infertile cannot, in most cases, administer fertility treatment to herself: she needs clinical assistance.

The question of whether a right demands positive action arises in a healthcare system such as the National Health Service in the UK, where treatment is free at the point of delivery and paid for indirectly through tax on income of the whole population. Decisions have to be made about what sorts of treatments can validly be offered and funded within such a health service (and by extension what sorts of research projects), and which treatments should be paid for at the point of delivery. Artificial reproduction is one such area; another is the operation to change one's sex; another, the removal of tattoos; another, some forms of plastic surgery. As skills to alter or restore the human condition proliferate, so does this list of treatments which are not related to saving lives but are related to well-being. The relevant question seems to be whether the conditions which give rise to the search for treatment, such as childlessness, discomfort with one's gender, or being ugly or unsightly in one's own eyes, can really be called disease or illness. But since there is so much disagreement over whether they are diseases or not, identifying that as the question does not help very much. It is easier to work on the basis that everyone has a duty merely to *let* P do X, though, as in the case of the errant child, there may be things we would feel it our duty not to let P do. It is nearly impossible to identify those things which we have a duty *actively to assist* P in doing, or even do for him. However, this sort of *laissez faire* response to rights is not much use to us if we cannot obtain what we want without help, such as having a child by artificial means.

(iii) **P has the power to do X.** This sort of right is gained by physical strength, or by powers conferred by the state, or other means. It could be argued that these are the only rights which have any practical use, for merely proclaiming rights, however logically valid they may be, does not help if a more powerful entity decides to ignore or override them. For example, to urge that we have a right to free speech, in a society whose government practises censorship, has little practical use. What we need is the means by which to exercise that right, that is, both the skill or ability to do the thing, and the power or freedom to exercise it. In the context of medical research, the significant power a patient needs is autonomy, that is, the ability to make decisions about and for herself. The question of autonomy will be considered in more detail, taking into account both the patient, who has to be competent to exercise her autonomy, and the doctor, who has to respect her autonomy so that she *can* exercise it.

(iv) **P has an immunity with regard to X:** We have no duty not to do X, and moreover no-one has the power to alter that situation. This fourth definition is meaningful in the legal context only: the constitution may grant us an immunity and no-one can take that immunity from us.

Interest theory and choice theory

Rights theories can be further elaborated by dividing them into choice theory and interest theory. Choice theory states that, apart from the right to liberty, we only have rights in so far as someone else has a duty towards us. Hence, Q makes a promise to P, and therefore has a duty to keep that promise. Because of the situation, P possesses a right, namely, the right to release Q from the promise. P's right is the correlative of Q's duty. However, as Waldron points out, I consider that I have a duty not to harm or maim other creatures, but I do not regard myself as released from that duty if the creatures tell me that I am free to maim and harm them. This observation is relevant to the question of whether or not it is ethical to conduct risky non-therapeutic research on consenting people.

Interest theory, elaborated, as it happens, by Jeremy Bentham, states that a right exists only where it is possible to say in advance who is the beneficiary of the duty, or whose interests are directly affected by the duty (Hart, 1973). Hence, the first example of the promise made by one person to another confers a right upon the promisee, but the second example of not harming other creatures confers no rights, the duties being too general and only indirectly related to particular individuals. Waldron argues that this theory of rights can be made to work if it is taken further than Bentham takes it. Rights can be identified which have no specified duty or indeed person whose duty it is, but which can nevertheless be acknowledged by a moral theory. For example, we may recognize that a baby in Somalia has a right to be fed, without knowing what the specific duty is that correlates with that right, nor knowing how that right is to be recognized in practice (such as who is going to meet the need). What such a recognition does is to identify towards whom duties may lie. The explication of the right is the appropriate ground for the assignment and allocation of duties. This sort of underlying right may incur any or all of the Hohenfeldian cluster of definitions; the choice of which will depend upon the right we are seeking to assert.

Choice theory is resonant of a kind of rights theory much in evidence before this century and not so much thereafter. This theory states that the only genuine right that exists is the right to liberty. The theory lent itself to minimalist, *laissez faire* government, which was merely required not to stand in the way of anyone exercising his liberty except in so far as it harmed others. It required no action to ensure that rights were upheld. On this account, socio-economic rights such as the right to free medical assistance, elementary education and a basic standard of living were regarded as debasing the language of rights and a category error. This century has seen a greater recognition of these services as rights, following the extended interest theory Waldron proposes. If we regard such services as medical assistance as a right, then active duties are demanded, if not of us, then of someone. If, on the other hand, we see only liberty as a right, no such activity is demanded, since all we have to do is not to intervene. So the problem lies with deciding what is ours by right, and what is not. If more rights than liberty are claimed, then interest theory has to be employed. If only liberty, then choice theory will suffice. One important consequence of this distinction is that under the choice theory of rights, only autonomous beings can have rights, because only autonomous beings are capable of exercising the liberty of choice that it then becomes our duty not to obstruct. Interest theory confers rights upon those without autonomy, such as the baby in Somalia. The task interest theory has, however, is to state what rights people do have other than liberty, and this, I admit, is impossible to do in any way which can be practical. This is the predicament the NHS faces in trying to decide what treatments people have a right to expect, free at the point of delivery. It is failing to suggest answers which are capable of rational defence, and often resource allocation decisions change with geography. Without a sound basis upon which to determine the rights it is proper to defend, interest theory is in danger of turning into Karl Marx's understanding of rights. He thought that rights separated people from their communities and bound them in their own private interests (Marx, 1843).

Choice theory of rights is capable of a more rational defence than interest theory. The mutual recognition of the right to liberty would go a long way towards according the respect that human beings should receive from each other, further, perhaps, than is clear at first sight, which sees only the *laissez faire* nature of the duties this right demands. If each one of our actions has an impact, the extent of which cannot be predicted, but which we assume goes further than we are able to see, respecting the liberty of (all) others demands unselfish behaviour even when we are alone. For example, taking more than we need of anything has an ultimate impact on the environment and ecological balance of the world. Demanding first place necessitates others taking second place.

Does the choice theory of rights have an answer to the problem of the Somalian baby? Interest theory gave us a reason for the duty to provide her with nourishment and shelter. It could be argued that the right to liberty is also sufficient for these purposes, if it is the taking of what is hers through selfishness and greed that has meant she cannot eat or find shelter, or rather her parents cannot. They have no difficulty in doing so, if given the basic tools (Yunus, 1998). The tools of subsistence need to remain with the baby's parents and not to be taken away by others for their own purposes, such as civil war or greedy Western markets. Her parents need this freedom to express their own potential in their own way, rather than patronage. In order to exercise their freedom, assistance may be needed and positive duties may therefore follow, such as providing the means to overcome the effects of natural disasters or civil war. But this can be seen as a duty to enable the right to freedom, not a duty to feed and clothe, even if food and shelter are offered as part of the assistance.

Of course, the right to liberty can be abused. It only works if we use it as a basis for respecting another's right to liberty, rather than trying to exercise our own. If the right is understood in the Marxist sense of giving us freedom to do what we want, it becomes licence and there is no constraint on the choices made. But if it is taken as a basis upon which to recognize the essential reasonableness and freedom in each person with whom we come into contact, and indeed those with whom we do not come into contact (who may nevertheless be affected by our actions), it forms a useful guide to conduct, which is what ethics is about. That is to say, we should not claim rights for ourselves, only respect them in others. This, in my view, is the ethical value of the language of rights.

The practical value of right-based deontological moral theory for the analysis of the ethics of research on humans, is that we should always consult the judgement of those who are affected by our actions. This specific version of rights theory I shall call right-based morality. In research on humans, right-based morality translates into the requirement to consult potential research participants before enrolling them into studies.

The validity of rights

The right that is in question as regards research on humans can be called the right to self-determination. That is, a person has the right to withhold consent from taking part in a research project, if she so wishes. Using the first definition of a right according to Hohenfeld, we might say that patients and people in general have a right *not* to take part in research. For this right to be defended, people may not only not become research participants if they do not want to, but also they may not become research participants by default, that is, their express permission needs to be sought before they are enrolled. Such is the current climate of opinion, particularly amongst research ethics committees, that this right tends to go unquestioned. But this was not always the fashionable view, and indeed is not a view shared by all researchers even today. If it is to be upheld, its validity needs to be demonstrated so that it can be defended even when the assumption of the primacy of autonomy goes out of fashion, as it may do in respect of, *inter alia*, organ donation.

In order to identify what underpins the right of a person to refuse to take part in research, we will consider the circumstances of a research project which is ethically acceptable according to goal-based and duty-based criteria. So, the research is aiming to answer an important question which can demonstrably be seen to be useful for future patients. It is therapeutic, and the risks to the research participants related to the taking of the experimental or control treatments are adequately balanced by their anticipated therapeutic benefits from it. Other risks from extra research procedures are minimal. The clinician conducting the research is certain that he is doing the right thing by his patient in putting her into the trial, because he genuinely does not know which of the treatments in the trial is better. Is anything ethical being left out of the decision whether or not to enrol his patient? The answer might be, that what is left out is any consultation of the wishes of the patient in the matter. But suppose the clinician thinks that it would unnecessarily distress and confuse his patient to be given a choice whether or not to take part in the research? The patient trusts the doctor; the doctor believes the trial is the best place for the patient; the trial is aiming at a beneficial goal. Is the doctrine of respect for autonomy sufficiently important to override even the duty-based concern that its application would possibly cause harm? The answer, I submit, is that autonomy *is* important enough. I return to the moral theory of Kant to explain why, and relate his philosophy to the choice theory of rights.

Kant's autonomy of reason

Like the Renaissance humanists, Kant equated reason and freedom, by which he meant that reason was free from 'natural grounds', 'sensuous impulses' and 'inclinations', and free from empirical conditions. Distinguishing it from the act of understanding, which is tied to the conditions of a possible experience, reason does not 'follow the order of things as they present themselves in appearance, but frames for itself with perfect spontaneity an order of its own according to ideas, to which it adapts the empirical conditions, and according to which it declares actions to be necessary, even though they have never taken place, and perhaps never will take place.' (Kant, 1787, p. 576). It is to this essential reasonableness in each human which respect for autonomy should rightly direct itself. Unless we give others the opportunity to exercise their own reason in coming to understand what they *ought* to do, we deny what is essentially human in them. This, together with the capacity to express their intelligence through the power of speech, is what distinguishes human beings from animals. Notice, however, that it is Kant's understanding of reason that is invoked as that which must be honoured through respect for autonomy. His understanding of reason is that it is capable of discovering what *ought* to happen. It is not an expression of personal desire, which Kant carefully separates from the exercise of pure reason. The right that is being defended in the context of research on humans is not the right to do whatever we please, it is the right demanded absolutely by the exercise of pure reason. The existence of this sublime quality permitted, the choice theory of rights is sufficient to support people's right to consent to participate in research. This is because if we did not seek their consent we would be denying them the liberty to decide to act according to their own reason, which, by its nature, Kant asserts, wills what is good.

This is an altogether higher notion of a right than has elsewhere been suggested. Often, as seen at the beginning of the chapter, rights are invoked as a way of protecting the weak against the strong, a notion investigated shortly. What I would suggest is that the purpose of seeking consent from people is not to protect them against stronger forces, but to give them an opportunity to exercise what makes them essentially human, pure reason, which is precisely *not* weak. It is asking, in our context, the clinician to respect that which is finest and most noble in human nature.

Kennedy's rights for the weaker party

Kant's language, and my own in the previous section, is high-flown. We may feel that discussions of pure reason are simply too idealistic and impractical. Ian Kennedy's analysis of patient rights is more down to earth. He has always argued that the appropriate basis for medical law is human rights, not just the rights which are declared in international and national charters and conventions, such as the Nuremberg Code, the Declaration of Helsinki and the International Declaration of Human Rights, but also the 'inchoate rights which are the product of reasoned moral analysis' (Kennedy, 1988, p. 386). Kennedy notes that talk of rights in the medical context has often provoked hostility from the medical profession or its spokespeople.

This is because the rights discussed are asserted as the rights of patients. Such assertions do not sit well with a profession which is, quite properly, educated to think of itself as concerned with the difficult task of caring for the sick and seeking to overcome illness. Talk of rights is often represented ... as if it inevitably involves ... strict or rigid restrictions on what the doctor may do.' (Kennedy, 1988, p. 386)

Recalling Hohenfeld's definitions of rights, it can be recognized that what is under threat is the 'privilege' right which doctors have traditionally enjoyed, and Kennedy points out that, after all, clinical freedom is itself a right. But there is a counterpart to the doctor's right to clinical freedom, argues Kennedy, which is the patient's right. It is the patient's right which sets the framework within which the doctor's discretion may be exercised. This right has a further contingent importance because:

As between the doctor and the patient there is an inevitable imbalance or disequilibrium of power. The doctor has information and skill which the patient, who lacks these, wishes to employ for his benefit. (1988, p. 387)

These powers possessed by the doctor include 'the privilege to touch and invade the body of the patient' (p. 387). Hence, insisting upon rights that accrue to the patient introduces a check on the privilege rights of the doctor, a check which comes from outside his own moral and professional framework, and which can, therefore, be judged independently of him on behalf of the patient.

Kennedy argues that the right that must be asserted above all is the right to respect for autonomy. The patient may not have the same power as the doctor by virtue of knowledge and experience, and she may be in the hands of the doctor as regards the receiving of the right treatment for her condition, but she does, or should, have the power to agree to what is to happen to her.

We could adopt the choice theory of rights, which was the most minimal of right-based theories, asking only that we respect another's liberty, to be the basis for patient autonomy. Or we could prefer the Kantian notion of the autonomy of reason as the appropriate basis. Or we could adopt Kennedy's view that it is to redress the imbalance of power between doctor and patient that requires this respect. In each case, I will conclude that autonomy should be respected, and that it can be respected by always seeking the patient's permission before doing anything to her.

Scarman's test

The Kantian definition of reason, namely, that in a person who is capable of making a good and right decision, is that which should be respected and referred to when seeking consent. It is not at all the same as consulting the personal inclination of a patient, which may be, for example, to avoid treatment which she ought to undergo for her own well being. What if, however, the reasoning of the patient does not concur with the reasoning of the doctor? If it always did, there would be no need to consult the patient, since she would always agree anyway. Respecting a person's autonomy requires consulting her, which implies that the patient may, for her own good reasons, disagree. Suppose then that the reasons are not, in the view of the doctor, good ones? Does that mean that the patient is not actually exercising her reason, but rather referring to something else, like her inclinations; or worse still, does it mean that the patient is not, in fact, competent to make a decision? Suppose the doctor was convinced that his patient's refusal, say, to receive a particular treatment, was based on flawed judgement? Should he conclude that his patient's autonomy is suspect, and override her? Or should he accept that there may be aspects to what is proposed which are unwanted by the patient for her own good reasons, which he is unaware of or does not understand? I suggest the doctor should take the latter course. Otherwise the principle of respect for autonomy becomes meaningless, since it only includes the exercising of that autonomy which furnishes similar views to those of the doctor.

The distinction between what the patient might regard as reasonable and right and what his doctor thinks was recognized by Lord Scarman in his judgement in the Sidaway case (1985). The question under discussion then was what level of risk it was right to inform the patient about, to which question I shall return in a moment. What is significant for the present argument is Lord Scarman's statement, that the determination of what should be told to the patient depended not upon what the doctor thought would be appropriate, but rather *a reasonable person in the patient's position*. Hence the focus was on the patient's view, not the doctor's. The judgement resonates with Kant's account of rational beings and their proper treatment, though it should be noted that this 'prudent patient' test does not focus on what the individual patient's view might be, but, rather, what a reasonable person would want.

However, to impose upon the doctor the rule of accepting his patient's views even when they disagree with his own may put impossible strains on his integrity, if the disagreement lies in situations which may require the doctor to do what he really believes to be wrong. The adoption of the choice rather than the interest theory of rights helps to distinguish between those circumstances where the doctor *must* accept the views of his patient, and those where he need not. It would be wrong to override the wishes of a patient when they consist merely in the refusal of a treatment the doctor thinks is right. But to respect the wishes of a patient who is *asking* for something the doctor believes is wrong is taking the rights of the patient too far, not least because the consequence of respecting that right would be to oblige the doctor positively to act in a way contrary to his own reason. This distinction is made, for example, in the explicit recognition of a doctor's right to refuse to help to procure, or to carry out, abortions. This right was reiterated at the 1999 British Medical Association Conference.

The applications of right-based thinking

In the context of medical research we are not faced with the situation of a patient asking for a treatment. We are concerned with cases where patients, or healthy people, will be asked to become research subjects. The right-based morality that I am going to adopt for the purpose of analysing the ethics of research on humans consists, then, in this: that we should consult the wishes of those most affected by our actions. I am also going to include the right of patients to have their confidentiality respected. This is a narrow definition of rights, but it is sufficient when taken together with the goal- and duty-based approaches to complete the analysis of the ethics of medical research on humans.

The consent procedure

For consent to be valid, it must be (i) given by a competent person; (ii) adequately informed; and (iii) voluntary.

Competence and the use of vulnerable groups in research
There will be times when potential research subjects have no competence, such as when they are unconscious, mentally incapacitated (though this is contentious), or too young to make a reasonable decision. Such cases cannot in fact be dealt with under our understanding of right-based morality since these people do not have the ability to express choice. However, these cases raise the consent issue in respect of who should be consulted if the patient cannot be.

Determining a child's competence

Children gain competence to different degrees and about different things over time. Some very young children, who suffer chronic medical conditions, may have a complete understanding of their situation, and be able to participate fully in any consent procedure. Others will be less comprehending. In the UK, the law recognizes this differentiation and offers what is known as the Gillick competence test to establish whether the child or her parents should be the ones to consent to treatment. The Gillick test arose out of a famous case (Gillick v Norfolk and Wisbech Health Authority, 1986) in which a mother took a Health Authority to court over the fact that a General Practitioner had prescribed contraceptives to her 15-year-old daughter without informing her. She eventually lost the case, which went all the way to the House of Lords, and the Gillick test emerged. It states that if, in the view of the clinician, the child is capable of understanding the nature and consequences of her treatment, that child is deemed competent and her consent overrides that of her parents. This ruling does not mention research, and I imagine that a court would expect a greater level of competence in order to validate a child's consent to research than to treatment. She might need to be able to understand randomization, altruism, or blind allocation of treatments, to name but a few of the concepts that arise in the research as distinct from the treatment context.

Decisions on behalf of an incompetent child or adult

Where a child is clearly incompetent, such as a baby, then the people *in loco parentis* are the ones whose consent has to be sought. But their consent can only be given to that which is in the best interests of the child. This, of course, is precisely what becomes the most relevant question in relation to any incompetent potential research subject. Interestingly, however, while it is the parent whose consent must be sought on behalf of an incompetent child, in the UK the law decrees that no one may consent on behalf of another adult. It is up to the person's doctor to decide what is in her best interests. As with parents deciding on behalf of their children, this process is not at all the same as the process of obtaining consent from the person who is the potential research subject. Right-based morality is about respecting the autonomy of the interested parties. It is about precisely *not* doing what we think is the best for another, but eliciting from her what she believes to be right for herself. Whether it is the researcher/doctor or a parent who has to make the decision on behalf of the incompetent patient, that decision will be made on her behalf, using best interest criteria. This is a duty-based moral decision, not a right-based one. The use of advance directives, made out before incompetence sets in, indicating patients' wishes, has increased the possibility of using right-based criteria to determine courses of treatment. Even advance directives may be disregarded, however, if it is the doctor's view that its requests are not in the patient's best interests.

When an incompetent adult or a child clearly needs treatment, it is given without consent, and its moral justification is duty-based: that is, it is in the patient's best interests that the treatment be given. If research is proposed involving incompetent subjects, the duty-based issue of best interests becomes the important deciding factor. In therapeutic research there is the equipoise test together with the consideration of whether the interests of the individual concerned would be best served by receiving treatment as a participant in a trial. Some would regard these criteria as sufficient to make it ethical to enrol an incompetent patient into a therapeutic trial. Others consider that any randomized controlled trial cannot, by definition, be said to be in each individual patient's best interests, since the treatment is not being tailored precisely to each individual. Non-therapeutic research on people who cannot consent is more difficult to justify, for non-therapeutic research cannot be said to be in the best interests of a research subject. If she is unable to consent to it on her own behalf then no moral justification for the research is left except the goal-based one of the desirable consequences. It can be the case that the only way important developments in some areas of medicine can be made is if non-therapeutic research on incompetent subjects takes place, for example, research into the causes of Alzheimer's disease. These can be the most difficult research projects about which to make ethical decisions, particularly when the goals seem very important. Examples of this will be discussed in Chapter Seven, where it emerges as a duty-based issue. Suffice it to say here that allowing such research to happen, even when the goals are extremely significant and the risks minimal, is no light matter, for the principles of behaviour demanded by duty- and right-based morality have perforce been compromised. It was the compromising of precisely these principles that made possible some of last century's worst excesses, starting with the notion that (some sorts of) people were expendable.

Competence in the ordinary adult

In the UK, as in many other countries, the law regards everyone over the age of 18 as competent unless there are compelling reasons not to, for example if the person is unconscious. In practice it is more accurate to say that there are degrees of competence even amongst those whom the law deems fully competent. In medicine, and medical research, patients are frequently not fully competent. This may be because of their illness, their medication, their physical circumstances or their emotional state. These factors encroach on a person's competence and cannot be ignored if the consent procedure is to be taken seriously. At the same time, the law's clear-cut approach reflects a Kantian notion of personal responsibility: that rational beings are answerable for their actions, so that even if someone does not feel very competent she should still try to make right decisions if called upon to do so, accept responsibility for what happens to her, and be willing to face the consequences of what she does decide.

Adequacy of information

In order for a patient to make a valid decision about whether or not to take part in research, she needs to comprehend information whose context is medicine. It takes several years for an individual to be trained sufficiently to call himself a doctor. Medical research is by its nature often at the vanguard of medical practice and so specialized that even qualified doctors can find it difficult to understand the nature and purpose of different research projects. There is evidence that concepts which are not found solely in the medical context, such as the concept of randomization, are not easily explained and understood (Snowdon et al., 1997). It is unlikely, then, that someone with no medical training is going to understand the detail of what is proposed. We can imagine taking time to inform a single individual whom we know well, tailoring the information-giving process to her particular needs and ability, but the research context demands giving information to hundreds, sometimes thousands, of people. I would not be wholly pessimistic about this process, provided those tasked with communication are aware of the challenges. The best teachers are the ones who, though experts in their subjects, are nevertheless able to convey the principles of their subject to schoolchildren. It has to be acknowledged, however, that the physical circumstances of many healthcare settings are not conducive to a genuinely informative exchange between a patient and her doctor.

Voluntary nature of the decision

Freedom to choose is the ultimate expression of autonomy. However, for the patient being asked to take part in research there are numerous influences affecting her freedom, related to: her condition, which may have an effect on his mental state; her location, which may be in the somewhat depersonalizing and dependent atmosphere of a hospital bed, in which, despite everyone's best efforts, she still feels she has to ask permission to do anything; and the all-important relationship with her doctor. It is this last factor which seems to me to count most against a free decision being made, for reasons which are not all bad. The doctor's powerful position in relation to his patient can give rise, not only to fear that the doctor will not be pleased if the patient does not agree to his requests, but also to trust, in that she will assume that the doctor will never ask her to do anything that is bad for her. She might, therefore, believe that there is no reason to refuse any request he might make. Therefore, the doctor *should* never ask his patient to do something which is harmful, whether it is in the interests of future patients or not. This would be counter to his *raison d'etre*, which is, after all, to heal, not to harm, but it does detract from the voluntary nature of any decision the patient may make.

Concluding remarks on consent

Although there are many obstacles to the success of the consent procedure, the need for it is still paramount, as the discussion in the first half of the chapter showed. Not respecting a patient's autonomy is equivalent to treating her as expendable. In Kant's terms, she should be treated as an end in herself, and never merely as a means to an end. According to Kennedy, not seeking consent leaves all the power in the hands of the doctor. He already has the advantage over his patient, in that he has more knowledge than his patient. Giving the doctor the freedom to act as he thinks best, without consulting his patient's wishes, doubly disadvantages the patient. The choice theory of rights, which is the most minimalist of rights theories, nevertheless places an obligation on the doctor to seek his patient's consent, because otherwise he will not be respecting her right to liberty.

For these reasons, we should not discard the consent procedure despite its practical difficulties. Rather, we should find ways to overcome them. It should be recognized, however, that in the medical context, there are some things which are too risky for doctors to ask their patients to face, even if, *particularly if*, the patient might agree if she *was* asked.

Confidentiality

Confidentiality is a right-based issue because it involves respecting that which is private to a person, which, if it cannot be said to belong to her, certainly does not belong to anyone else. This is information of a personal nature, which is disclosed only on the understanding that it will be kept confidential, as is the case in the medical encounter between patient and doctor. There are numerous cases of research where confidentiality is threatened or compromised, one of which will be discussed in Chapter Eight. The principle is simple: if a patient speaks to her doctor about her private medical life she does so on the express understanding that her doctor, if he does pass the information on, will only do so to those who have a direct responsibility for her healthcare.

Consent to the disclosure of private information to those with direct responsibility for the patient's healthcare may be inferred and need not be explicitly sought. However, a doctor cannot infer his patient's consent to her identifiable medical information being made available to researchers, who do not have a direct interest in her medical care. If such disclosure were to be made, it would be a violation of the right-based demand to respect a person's privacy. It would not be justifiable on duty-based grounds either, since it is not in a person's best interests that her records are disclosed. The reasons for doing it (and they are often compelling) would be goal-based. For example, the national incidence of a particular disease plays an important part in the planning and delivery of the right kinds of health care. The information about this is gathered by epidemiologists, who will search patient records for it. Sometimes thousands of records are involved. Seeking consent from each patient before looking non-therapeutically at their records would honour the right-based principle of respecting autonomy, but it would also render the research impossible logistically and financially. So, currently, such research is conducted without patient consent. In the UK, as elsewhere, researchers are bound not to disclose medical information to any other source (Department of Health, 1996), but they themselves have access to it. Another example is of researchers seeking a particular patient population for the purposes of their research, for example, all people in a particular area who are recently bereaved for research into bereavement recovery rates. These researchers may find out lists of such patients from GPs and then approach the potential recruits directly, potentially causing tremendous upset. Also, there are an increasing number of disease registers from which researchers can obtain information about particular patient groups with a given disease, thus avoiding asking GPs. If those patients whose details are on such registers do not know they are listed there, there was a breach of confidence when the patients' name and details were entered on the register (not at the point when the researcher gains access to the information). One of the reasons for creating disease registers is to make such information easily accessible for valid purposes, and no doubt patients with conditions which would benefit from more research would welcome better organization of such information, were they to be asked. The ethical problem arises because of doing it without asking first.

These examples of breaches of confidentiality are instances where goal-based and right-based claims to determine what is morally right come into conflict with each other. As with the dilemma over non-therapeutic research on incompetent subjects, it is essential that researchers, if they choose to go ahead with such research, and research ethics committees, if they choose to approve the research, recognize the cost of achieving the goal in terms of the loss of deontological principle. On the other hand, the harm to patients whose records are used in this way is negligible. It could even be argued that there is *no* harm, if the patients never know that researchers have been allowed to see their records. Meanwhile, the advantages of records-based research are numerous. This sort of research sets goal-based moral values at loggerheads with duty- and right-based ones. Solutions, therefore, will always be unsatisfactory to some people.

Summary and concluding remarks

This chapter has considered four different accounts of rights: the Hohenfeldian cluster of rights, which helped to clarify what the word 'right' can mean
in different contexts; Waldron's distinction between choice and interest
theories of rights, where interest theory demanded positive duties and choice
theory demanded respect for people's liberty; Kant's elucidation of the
autonomy of reason and its consequent requirement that all rational beings
be treated as ends in themselves; and finally, Ian Kennedy's assertion that
when there is an imbalance of power in a relationship the weaker party must
be granted rights which place strict constraints on what the stronger party
may do. In the context of medical research on humans, the practical recognition of rights lies in the seeking of consent from any potential research
participant, and also in respecting her confidentiality.

The three factors that make up the consent procedure are that the person
whose consent is sought be competent, adequately informed, and able to
make her choice voluntarily. Competence is absent in some people, in which
cases the duty-based demand that they are treated in their best interests takes
precedence. If a child, her parents must consent or refuse according to, again,
her best interests. Competence may be compromised by states of health, but
it has to be assumed to be there in people over the age of 18, and sometimes
younger, for the purposes of the consent procedure. Information can be
difficult to convey. Finally, the choice needs to be voluntarily made, and this
may be affected by the way the patient relates to her doctor.

These obstacles to success do not mean that consent should not be sought.
Rather, they indicate that it is unwise to rely upon the consent procedure to
validate the ethics of a research project on its own. Hence, the right-based
approach to moral thinking is, like goal- and duty-based thinking, necessary
but not sufficient for the purpose of ensuring that research is ethical. Nevertheless, even if the seeking of consent is not the only important ethical
principle to uphold in research on humans it is still crucially important, as
the earlier part of this chapter showed. The analysis of the process of
obtaining consent emphasised the point that a researcher should only seek
consent to do things which are right, as far as he is able to determine. Hence,
the goal-based demand that the research be aimed at something good and
important must be met first, then the duty-based demand that no inappropriate harm should befall the research participants who take part should be
met, and then finally, the patient's wishes must be consulted. These three
components, based on the three approaches to morality, all play their part in
providing a framework for determining the morality of a research project
involving human participants.

There are some sorts of research projects which violate right-based moral
claims. Research on incompetent participants, and research which involves

breaching confidentiality, are both examples of this. In these situations, even deciding not to conduct the research on the grounds of caution is morally problematic, for it means that goal-based moral claims are ignored. In the second part of the book cases will be encountered where the three approaches come into conflict with each other, and we will see whether it will be possible to come to resolutions that do sufficient justice to all three approaches.

5

From principles to practice

Introduction

This chapter acts as the link between the three theoretical chapters and the three practical chapters. Until now the three approaches to moral questions have been discussed in the context of human participant research at the level of ideas and theoretical applications. In the next three chapters cases will be analysed using the three approaches. The same order of presentation will be followed. Each chapter will focus on one of the three approaches, and the practical issues discussed will mirror those raised within each of the theoretical chapters. This introductory chapter will summarize the philosophical foundations of each of the three approaches, and introduce the cases to be discussed in the second half of the book.

Goal-based morality

Goal-based morality's theoretical basis summarized

Chapter Two introduced goal-based morality, describing the theories of some of its more famous utilitarian forbears. Utilitarianism considers the outcome of an action to be its moral determinant, rather than the content of the action itself. In simple terms, this means working out the extent to which an action maximizes happiness. Jeremy Bentham thought that each person affected by an action should count as one, so that the more people who were made happy by an action, the more justified it was. This simple theory, although attractive because it requires no complex moral code or belief in a higher authority, nevertheless countenances and even justifies harm to some. It does not seek to condemn any action whatsoever, if it maximizes happiness.

In response to this accusation of being open to justifying bad acts for predicted good consequences, rule utilitarianism was proposed. In this theory, rules are applied which are utilitarianly justified: if followed, they will lead to the greatest happiness for the greatest number. Although this is a more acceptable moral theory because it opens the way to outlawing certain morally abhorrent acts, it has lost the simplicity that had made utilitarianism attractive in the first place. For the rules have to be devised prior to particular actions being proposed. With act utilitarianism, as Bentham's utilitarianism is known, the situation is real and the consequences of an action easier to foresee. With rule utilitarianism, the situations are anticipated and their consequences hypothetical. Hence an authority has to be recognized. Where are the rules to come from, if not from tradition, belief and even religion? R.M. Hare, for example, a rule utilitarian, finds his rules in the Christian commandment to love God and neighbour.

In any case, if we are hard-headed utilitarians, are we not required to perform that act which maximizes happiness, regardless of the content of the act, because we are not supposed to mind if moral rules from tradition or religion are broken? Utilitarianism has an inherent debasing pull, as Williams has pointed out, in that, being by nature pre-emptive, it countenances actions which, taken in themselves, are fairly nasty, in order to avoid what are perceived as worse consequences. In medical research, the more important the goal, the more the claims of duty- and right-based morality will be under threat. However, not to consider the consequences of a research project as part of the ethical analysis would be literally nonsensical, since research is always undertaken to achieve a goal.

Goals of research in theory and practice

It is, therefore, important to consider whether the consequences of a research project are good and desirable, even if they do not, finally, justify the action. This moral approach, adopted as just one part of the overall moral analysis, I called goal-based morality. In research, this involves considering the goals of the research in relation to their contribution to health care. Once it is clear what the research is aiming to do, the way in which it is carried out can be described, and then subjected to the scrutiny of duty- and right-based moral questions. Deciding what is a proper goal for research is not easy. How should research priorities be set? The possible goals a researcher might embark upon a research project to achieve are many, ranging from open-ended scientific curiosity to the promise of financial gain, with the gamut of answers to a variety of research questions in between. The challenge of goal-based morality is to find a reference point for the moral validity of the research goal. This attempt raises fundamental questions of what medicine should really be trying to achieve. I suggested that the ideal that researchers should hang on to is that of discovering complete cures in their medical fields which have no side effects. This provides an ultimate goal towards which all research can ultimately aim, even though the everyday reality is that research takes steps on the way to it.

In Chapter Six, where actual cases are discussed by way of illustration of issues in goal-based morality, organ transplantation is taken as a case study. The procedure for organ transplantation involves harm in several different forms, which research is continually seeking to remedy with improvements and refinements. In particular, different sources for organs are being investigated. So far, no method has been achieved which does not convey harm in one form or another. But the future holds new possibilities for safer, better treatment.

Research method summarized

Once the goal of the research has been identified, the appropriate method for achieving it has to be chosen. As described in Chapter Two, this might be a randomized controlled trial, in which groups of patients are randomly allocated the treatments which are being tested, and both researchers and participants are masked to avoid bias. The method chosen might be observational, with no experimental intervention. Or it might be qualitative, seeking to elicit the views of the researched with no imposition of the researcher's beliefs on the study or its results.

The practical implications of the choice of research method

Once the appropriate method has been chosen, it is important to let the science speak and not to superimpose beliefs, however rational they might seem, on to the evidence. The importance of this discipline is demonstrated in the two cases related to research method that are discussed in Chapter Six. One, a historical example, is the discovery of penicillin. This story shows the consequences of holding particular notions of how the world works. Penicillin was not properly discovered until old ideas about the immune system and the effectiveness of drugs had been dropped. A modern example of research into homeopathic medicines is then considered. The literature indicates that similar prejudices are standing in the way of clinicians being able to see the implications of the results of the research.

Summary of the problems with disseminating the results of research

Chapter Two said that disseminating the results of research is an intrinsic part of the research process. It then considered the obstacles which lay in the path of such dissemination. These were, first, that encouraging clinicians to put evidence into practice is not easy, because of ignorance of the research, unreasonable intransigence, or because the evidence is not sufficiently persuasive. Second, it is difficult to collect the right evidence together, because of publication bias (which might include not wanting to publish because the research was conducted unethically), because of researchers' and their sponsors' wish not to share results, and because the findings in published original papers needs to be supplemented by the correspondence which follows, and this is not often cited. Third, dissemination of results is part of the wider aim of encouraging evidence-based medicine, which often only deals with quantifiable results, and therefore might miss important, non-quantifiable aspects of medical practice.

Introduction to practical examples of dissemination problems

Chapter Six discusses, by way of illustration, research into so-called futile treatment, the results of which are to many minds morally unacceptable. It then briefly discusses pharmaceutical company research which found itself the result it wanted by dint of extended 'fishing'. Then some research into fetal monitoring during labour is mentioned, which produced results of statistical significance which were of no use to women in labour, nor to their babies.

   This third aspect of goal-based morality in research seems to undermine the first two, for what is the point of believing the research evidence if it is beset with problems? However, the examples are meant to be cautionary, not discouraging. They emphasize the need to ensure that the goal with which the research endeavour begins is really the one that is called for by reference to patients' needs and not serving some smaller aim. The problem with the three cases discussed under dissemination of results in Chapter Six was that the research question with which they began was misguided.

Duty-based morality

Duty-based morality's theoretical basis summarized

Chapter Three described two formulations of duty-based deontological morality. One is the tradition of natural law ethics, and the other is Kant's autonomy of reason giving rise to the categorical imperative. Natural law seeks to give an account of the world which provides a basis upon which to establish moral behaviour. The thesis is that everything has a natural function, and works according to that function. The natural way to live is the right way to live, and this can be discovered by investigating the way the natural world works. The difficulties with this thesis are that all definitions of 'natural' are open to question, and that equating what is natural with what is right can be nonsensical or illogical. However, the example given was that of the law of gravity. We cannot break the law, but we can ignore it. In ignoring it we suffer the consequences. That a doctor has a duty to act in her patients' best interests is true in the same way that the law of gravity is true. 'Natural' and 'right' are uncontentiously identical in this case. Moreover, the effect of following that natural law is good. The other formulation of duty-based morality is from Kant, who argues that, nature having endowed us with reason, we are bound to live dutifully, according to the moral law, rather than seek our own happiness. Reason is autonomous in that it can determine what is absolutely true by its own light, and not by virtue of some other agency which will be unreliable because of being external. Reason seeks to direct the will by means of the moral law. The moral law is formulated by Kant as the categorical imperative, that is, it must be obeyed by the precepts of reason. The categorical imperative is to act only according the maxims that can become universal laws, and only if we can consistently will that those maxims governing our actions should become universal laws.

The practical implications of duty-based morality

The application of duty-based morality for the purposes of medical research on humans is to be found in the way doctors/researchers should treat their patients/participants. As doctors, they must act in their patients' best interests. In therapeutic research, which is conducted in the context of medical care, the patients who are the research participants must be treated in the trial at least as well as they would be treated outside the trial. For this to happen, doctors must be in what I have called strong equipoise. Strong equipoise is the state of mind whereby doctors do not know which of two or more treatments being offered in a trial is best for their patients, and are therefore happy that their patients' best interests are served if they are randomly allocated to any one of them. Duty-based morality would also require that doctors should consider each of their patients as individuals with specific needs when deciding whether or not to enrol them in their research, and that the research is designed in such a way that researching doctors can continue to treat each participant in his best interests.

Introduction to examples

If a trial has amongst its treatment options a placebo arm, that is, the possibility that a participant may receive no treatment, that must also be accounted for in the doctors' state of equipoise. So they must be happy that their patients might receive only dummy treatments. This can present problems, discussed in theory in Chapter Three. The inclusion of a placebo arm in a trial is scientifically very important, as it adds to the rigour of the trial and makes the data easier to interpret, which is a goal-based imperative. And yet it can be directly counter to the doctor's duty of care. Chapter Seven discusses the issue of placebo-controlled trials in considerable detail, using several examples, for it is an issue that is likely to continue to vex researchers and research ethics committees for as long as trials using randomization continue. It is a good example of where duty-based and goal-based moral requirements come into conflict, where different people will be arguing an ethical line and yet disagreeing with each other.

Another situation in which duty-based morality comes into conflict with goal-based morality is in non-therapeutic research, in which there is no intention to benefit the research participants. In this situation of no benefit, there may still be risk of harm. Medical science may need to find an answer to certain questions, and future patients may benefit from the answer being known, and yet this cannot, as mentioned in the discussion of goal-based morality, be the sole justification for using people as research participants, especially as they may be harmed. The general rule given in most guidelines for research (Foster, 1997) is that non-therapeutic research should expose participants to no greater than minimal risk. This is something of an arbitrary measure, and of course different views will be held about what constitutes minimal risk. Chapter Seven discusses a controversial trial in which babies were placed in tents with 15% oxygen, to mimic the atmospheric conditions of an intercontinental flight, in an attempt to investigate a possible cause of sudden infant death syndrome. The research was thoroughly debated from an ethical point of view before it commenced, and its publication was hedged about by ethical commentaries. Nevertheless, the research went directly against the tenets of duty-based morality.

Duty-based morality also clashes with right-based morality when research participants, fully competent and healthy, agree to take part in research projects which will lead to harm, sometimes fatally so. This can and has been the case with healthy volunteer research, which is also discussed in Chapter Seven. Healthy volunteer research usually takes the form of Phase I studies of novel chemical agents. These agents, not yet called medicines, are given for the first time to humans to measure toxicity and pharmacokinetics, before being tried out in the patients for whom they are ultimately intended. Researchers perform medical examinations on the often young and impecunious students who volunteer to participate, in order to ensure that they are in a fit state to be research participants. However, not everything can be discovered by means of medical examinations, and the researchers rely on truthful accounts by the volunteers of their alcohol and drug use, and other potentially dangerous activities or states of health. The right-based view is that these volunteers, being competent and informed, can and should be relied upon to take care of their own welfare. The cases discussed in Chapter Seven indicate otherwise, offering a useful illustration of the conflict between duty-based and right-based morality which can arise in healthy volunteer research.

The principle that the doctor/researcher has a duty to benefit and not to harm her patients is what underlies the concern to uphold duty-based morality. Like the tremendous importance of the goal of the research being chosen rightly, so the doctor's duty to care needs to be retained at all times. If a research method demands a compromise of the doctor's duty, it is the science which should change, not the duty.

Right-based morality

Right-based morality's theoretical basis summarized

Chapter Four contained an account of some different theories of rights which have been used in moral philosophy, to underpin a discussion of the place of rights in medical research on humans. Several accounts of rights were considered. Choice Theory, the articulation of the right to freedom, was taken as one helpful way to think about rights for our purposes, together with Kant's description of human reason. In these terms, seeking consent to participate in research is an appeal to the rational aspect of a person, who will thereby make the best decision for all concerned. It is not a consultation of mere whims and fancies. Another way of thinking about rights which was discussed in Chapter Four is that proposed by Ian Kennedy, in which the articulation of the patient's rights takes the position of power away from the doctor and equalizes the relationship between doctor and patient. Expressed as the patient's consent to treatment (research, for our purposes), rights give patients the final say as to what is to happen to their body. Their consent to participation is the gatekeeper of the actions of the doctor.

Introduction to examples

However, there are difficulties with the process of obtaining consent, which were identified in Chapter Four. Chapter Eight gives those difficulties sub- stance by reference to a number of empirical studies, such as the one which showed considerable confusion about the concept of randomization amongst parents of neonates in a research project. Other empirical studies discussed investigate whether seeking consent gives rise to greater anxiety, which if true would be a duty-based reason for being wary of seeking consent. Yet more studies indicate that the consent process reduces recruitment rates of subjects for research, which threatens research. This, of course, is a goal-based con- cern, and provides a goal-based reason for being reluctant to take the consent process seriously. These threats to the claim of right-based morality, that seeking consent is of paramount importance, are not inconsiderable, which is why it is necessary to be able to give substance and weight to the principle that is elucidated in Chapter Four.

Chapter Eight also discusses research which cannot take place if consent is sought, when the outcome of the research would be affected if patients knew they were research participants. This represents a clash between goal-based and right-based morality. The case used for illustration was published in the *British Medical Journal*. In passing, the issue of whether research which has been conducted unethically should be published is discussed. Publishing it arguably provides an opportunity for something good to come out of something bad, but it also tacitly encourages bad practice. The discussion on consent is finished by ruminating on the status of written consent, and some empirical evidence for the way it is perceived by patients is offered.

Confidentiality is treated as a right-based issue in this analysis, and its importance and philosophical underpinning were described in Chapter Four. Chapter Eight discusses the case of records-based research, in which compelling goal-based arguments for conducting this sort of research without consent compete with right-based arguments for respecting patient confidentiality.

Does the three-approaches framework succeed?

Chapter Nine contains a discussion of the success of the three-approaches model for considering the ethics of medical research on humans. In this chapter I admit that the approach is by no means fool-proof. The role of research ethics committees is also discussed, as is the importance of researchers taking full moral responsibility for the research they propose to conduct. To demonstrate this point, the story of the way research has been governed in this country from the Nuremberg Code of 1947 until now is told. Step by inevitable step, the governance of research on humans has become increasingly regulated and restricted, bound by that voracious question, Who guards the guardians? Given that we cannot ultimately rely on others to guard and protect our own morality, there remains an imperative for each individual to take to heart, which is to take full moral responsibility for his own actions. The book ends with a plea and a guide for this.

6

Case studies of goal-based issues

Introduction

This chapter will cover specific cases of research whose goals, scientific methods and dissemination of results create particular and interesting ethical problems. As an example of ethical problems in research goals we will look at the aims of different branches of organ transplantation research. In seeking to improve the chances of people who are in need of new organs, tissue and skin, research moves in such ethically sensitive areas as elective ventilation, xeno-transplantation and the use of embryos as a therapeutic tool. When we come, secondly, to look at issues in research method, two examples will be considered. The first is the discovery of penicillin, and the second is research into homeopathic treatments. The two accounts have some similarities. Thirdly and finally the dissemination of results will be discussed, looking specifically at cases which highlight the difficulties in making evidence-based medicine a reality. These are: research into administering cardio-pulmonary resuscitation to neonates to determine whether and when that treatment is futile; research into uses for interferon; and research into fetal monitoring during labour.

Goals of research

When this issue was discussed in Chapter Two, it was suggested that re-searchers should aim at discovering treatments that cure without harm to individual patients or to the wider environment. The development of treat-ments for those whose organs are in disrepair and need replacing will now be taken as a case study of research goals.

Organ transplantation

Initial fears about Frankenstein's monster were overcome as, in the case of some organs at least, successful transplantation and the good quality of life of the recipients were demonstrated many times over. The outcomes of organ transplant operations continue to improve as more is understood of the treatment of what is called 'graft versus host disease', which is the problem of the recipient's immune system developing resistance to the donor's organ. A balance has to be struck between the immuno-suppressive drugs the host must take, to help her body accept the alien organ, and the need for the host's immune system to be allowed to continue to work against other disease insults. This is more-or-less successful in different bodies and with different organs. The receipt of an organ makes the difference between a person having a disease which is incompatible with life, and one which is compatible with life. That is to say, organ transplantation is not a cure even though it is life-saving. Hence, one of the qualifications for receiving an organ is that the patient must agree to adhere to the drugs regimen and life-style requirements that go with having someone else's organ in her body. Research in all the different aspects of organ transplantation is geared towards the successful receipt and carrying of a foreign organ. Both in terms of the overall goal and the individual parts of the different research projects that serve that goal, there remains little that is thought to be ethically questionable here.

Two areas remain of concern in organ donation from dead bodies. The first is the respect that is owed to the dead. It might seem irrational to think in terms of harm when removing organs from cadavers, but certain other practices raise questions about it. When we honour the dead, at a funeral or cremation, or at a service of commemoration, such as of those who died in a war, the focus of our attention is the body which is committed for burial or cremation, or the graveyard where those who fell were buried. Even now, the crematoria of the dead of World War One in Northern France and Belgium are tended with supreme care, and still visited by thousands who, to judge by the comments they write in the crematorium registers, are profoundly affected by what they find there. The commemoration is not, of course, of dead bodies; it is of the acts and qualities of the people who inhabited them. Nevertheless, respecting the physical remains is a way of showing respect for the person whose body it was. In the light of this, it must remain at least a concern that transplant surgeons have to harvest organs from bodies for therapeutic purposes. The furore caused when it becomes widely known that organs and other body parts have been taken without permission is symptomatic of the concern and sensitivity of the issue.

The second area of concern is the shortage of organs for donation. As the techniques for organ transplantation refine and the number of patients who qualify for transplantation increases, so the waiting lists for donors grow longer. The terrible choice has to be made as to who should qualify for an organ. Intelligent systems for keeping the allocation of organs fair have been devised. For example, in the UK, hospitals where organ transplantation is carried out are maintained on a rotating list. Great Ormond Street Hospital for Sick Children, where paediatric transplants are carried out, always remains in second place. So the availability of organs is based on chance, but it is a fair chance, and children are given high priority. The decision about which patients' names should be put on waiting lists requires a deliberate decision, however. Clinicians worry about the criteria they use for inclusion on the waiting lists. Should psychological factors play a part? What if a patient is eager for the transplant and yet has a history of non-adherence to medical regimens? What if her family does not seem sufficiently enthusiastic to provide the support she is going to need after surgery? Attempts to rationalize criteria for inclusion have failed at a national level, though they are made in individual hospitals, or by individual surgeons. Some surgeons, for example, believe that people with Down's Syndrome should not be offered the heart–lung transplant they often need, for the consequentialist reasons that they are going to die (relatively) young anyway, and that the prolonged life a transplant gives them only stretches out the time society has to support them, as they cannot be independent. Moreover, it is argued, their quality of life diminishes rapidly, for social rather than medical reasons, once they leave the protected environment of school and enter the adult world. Where a heart–lung transplant is needed and is not given, survival beyond school age is unlikely. This harsh view is counterbalanced by numerous successful projects of self-supporting communities of people with Down's Syndrome. Every criterion for exclusion can have such a countervailing argument.

I would argue that these sorts of decisions are essentially qualitative and subjective. They are not amenable to checklists, however much fairer that may seem. Each individual coming for consideration will have her own unique set of circumstances. Difficult as it is, it is far better that the decision is made on the basis of the person who is actually standing in front of the clinician, to whom he brings his experience and judgement, rather than by reference to some pre-arranged code.

Needless to say, constant efforts are made to increase the number of organs available for donation. The number of card-carrying donors remains small; the debate about whether to create an opt-out system of donation, whereby a person's organs are available unless that person has specifically requested otherwise, is alive and flourishing. It is a goal-based answer to the problem, which does not recognize the duty- and right-based moral obligations not to take organs from cadavers unless permission is specifically given.

Maintaining the condition of donor organs

Organs to be used for transplant need to be in a healthy condition. From the moment blood ceases to circulate in an organ it begins to deteriorate rapidly. If a brain-dead patient is kept on life support, then the organs remain vascularized as the blood continues to circulate around her body. It effectively means that a body (person?) is kept breathing and its or her heart beating for the purposes of harvesting good-quality organs. Although the utilitarian justification for it is considerable, the action taken on its own is 'fairly nasty' (Williams, 1993). An account by a medical student who witnessed the process performed on a young boy who had died in an accident is offered here. The process took place when the student was not yet used to such procedures and therefore saw it as a lay person would in the same circumstances.

Finally we were ready. After a few hours of work, the key moment was at hand. The anaesthetist turned off the ventilator and removed the machines supplying the heart with medications that were helping it to beat. The surgeon instructed Paul [another medical student] and me to feel the 'dying heart'. At the time, it felt no different from any other beating heart; it looked strong and healthy and had a regular motion. Then the arterial clamps were placed, and the vessels that connected the liver to the rest of the body were severed. The surgeon lifted the liver out of the body and rushed it to the waiting basin of an ice-cold solution especially designed to maintain it for as long as possible.

I marvelled at the powerful actions taking place before my eyes. The surgeon had taken a knife to another person's skin and was hoisting the internal organs into the air for all of us to see. I was reminded of an ancient religious ritual in which one life was sacrificed for the good of the rest of the community. Such patterns were repeating themselves here in the modern era.

Instead of following the surgeon's hands as she moved to take the kidneys, I was drawn back to the heart. In the minute after the machines were turned off, the boy's heart rate had slowed substantially. I could not help staring at the fading, barely beating muscle.

The flurry of activity continued as the kidneys were placed in their proper cold preservative. The surgeon's attention moved to the pancreas. At this point, the anaesthetist politely and uncomfortably excused herself after verifying that her tasks were finished. She could do nothing else for this patient. As she stood up to leave, I found my eyes again drawn to the heart. Now each beat was followed by a number of seconds of stillness. The boy had been dead for 16 hours, but all of my instincts were telling me that this was the moment, this was when Mark was really dying. I was standing next to the cloth that separated the surgical team from Mark's face. Because of the apparatus keeping the boy's chest open, the drape over his face was very close to the surgical field in which all of the action was taking place. When I looked to the head of the operating table, I could make out the outline of the boy's face under the cloth.

From there, my eyes were again drawn towards the open chest, and I saw Mark's heart beat in its final contraction. I found myself crying uncontrollably, my tears hidden from the people around me by my protective goggles and mask. The surgeons were too busy organising and removing tissue to notice or acknowledge my reaction. I felt as if I was the only one at the table who had witnessed Mark's passing; the others were caught up in the removal of organ after organ. The heart was finally taken from the chest as the person from the eye bank came to procure the eyeballs. (Rothstein, 1995).

I should point out that there are very few medical or surgical procedures that have no gruesome aspects to them. People tolerate them, both in themselves and in society as a whole, because of the hoped-for benefits. In most surgery, of course, the benefits accrue to the one whose body is being invaded. In the case of elective ventilation and organ harvesting, the benefits accrue to the recipients of the organs. This does not constitute an argument against the practice. The circumstances are that there is a shortage of organs, and though the dead body can be disrespected, the person who formerly occupied it cannot be harmed. That makes it better, on balance, to harvest organs from dead bodies rather than not to. But it is not the ideal solution even on its own terms, because of graft versus host disease, and because there are never enough organs to go around.

Xenotransplantation

The animal kingdom provides a further source of organs. The goal of research in xenotransplantation is to provide, successfully, animal cells, tissues and organs for humans. Research is currently focused on the use of pig organs, although the organs of old world monkeys and apes would be better tolerated by humans. The medical problems and risks of xenotransplantation, to which I shall briefly give some attention, are of three kinds: physiological; immunological; and microbiological (Weiss, 1998).

Physiological obstacles to the success of xenotransplantation as far as pig hearts are concerned are not considerable. The pig heart should be capable of functioning in a human body, even though it will have to pump blood upwards, to which it will be unaccustomed. But pig kidneys have a different structure and function from human ones, and may not function properly in the human body, chiefly because porcine erythropoietin, a hormone synthesized by the kidneys which is essential for regulating the production and maturation of red blood cells, does not act like human erythropoietin. There may, thinks Weiss, be many other physiological discordances which complicate the acceptance of the porcine kidney in the human body.

Immunological complications between pig and human are greater than those seen in the transfer of human organs into human bodies, because the graft of the animal organ can be destroyed in several different ways, all of which have to be prevented if the organ is to succeed in its new environment. The length of time and extent to which recipients of animal organs will have to remain on immuno-suppressive drugs to avoid rejection is not known. Such drugs have a deleterious effect on the body's capacity to remain protected from other insults, and the balance between taking sufficient immuno-suppressive drugs to prevent the organ being rejected, and taking doses which are small enough to ensure that the body is able to ward off other infections, is difficult enough to achieve with human organ donation. Porcine organs may need a much greater suppression of the immune system.

Microbiological risks from animal transplantation could be great. The risk of viruses lethal to humans being introduced into the human environment is present. Once the physical barriers to animal viruses are broken by the placing of animal tissue in the human body, there is a danger that the immuno-suppressive drugs, taken by the human to prevent rejection of the organ, will help a virus to propagate and adapt to its new host. There may also be viruses which are found to be lethal to humans which would have been quite harmless to the pig whose organs have been used. Herpes virus B of macaques only gives the monkeys cold sores but causes fatal encephalitis in humans. The same pattern may be seen in the transfer of porcine viruses. Of course, if the pigs could be reared in environments which keep them free from all viruses, this last risk should not be present.

There are, clearly, serious medical problems which stand in the way of successful xenotransplantation and much more research needs to be done to ensure that the risk to the human recipients is minimized. There are also wider implications of risk to the community in releasing unknown diseases. Weiss argues that the decision to receive an animal organ is based on a risk–benefit analysis. The risk is not just to the individual receiving the organ, who might be very willing to be so exposed if the alternative is death, but also to the community which may then become susceptible to hitherto unknown diseases. Weiss says this is just like the problem of taking antibiotics, the extensive use of which has led to substantial resistance in some bacteria, which has meant that the population is now exposed to more serious risk of infection than before. Individuals needing antibiotics to cure an infection may be willing to take the risk of future resistance, but they have something to gain from taking the antibiotics. The general population faces the same risks but not the immediate benefit. In this respect, xenotransplantation research is an example of a research goal that may cause harm at a more general level. This is not a sufficiently strong argument to suggest that the research should not take place, only that it is not a final answer.

Another, wider ethical question about xenotransplantation relates to the fact that the source of the tissue for transplantation is a living creature, which humans as a species have considerable responsibility not to harm. The argument for using pigs instead of apes and old world monkeys is that the primates would have to be born by caesarean section and brought up entirely apart from other monkeys, a condition which would, to a primate, be very cruel. Pigs, it is thought, perhaps mistakenly, can be reared in such conditions without the same cruelty being wrought. Although it is clear that different animals have different requirements for their welfare, and those of the primate are more complex than those of the pig, nevertheless it seems to me that the difference is only a matter of degree. Either way, the animal is being produced as a crop for harvesting. This dilemma is no different from the one in which animals are grown in order to be killed and eaten; which is, after all, the specific reason pigs are reared. There is also a question about whether xenotransplantation is just too unnatural, and that because of that, it is bound, in the end, to fail. Although I do not propose to defend or attack these lines of argument, I recognize that they introduce a question mark over the research goals in xenotransplantation. Therefore, again, if it were possible to find a different way of helping people whose organs are in need of repair, which did not involve such calculated growing and harvesting of organs in pigs, it would be better to use it.

Autografting using cloned embryos

One such way that is currently being researched is the development of autografting techniques, whereby a person, in effect, provides her own tissue and organ replacements. For this to be possible, however, the stem cells which grow in the early stages of embryo development have to be gathered. It is these cells which can be manipulated to grow into different tissues and organs. In order to grow and harvest stem cells, embryos have to be created. The technique for doing this is identical to the cloning process. The nucleus of a somatic adult cell of the human whose tissue is to be grown is transplanted into an unfertilized egg whose own nucleus has been removed. To put a quite remarkable process in extremely simple terms, the transfer of a nucleus, together with the introduction of some electricity, tricks the egg into thinking it has been fertilized. It then grows as an embryo from which stem cells can be harvested.

Research in this area is in its very early stages. The UK government asked the Human Fertilization and Embryology Authority and the Human Genetics Advisory Committee to submit to it a report on cell nuclear transfer and human cloning generally. The report (HFEA/HGAC, 1998) argued that whilst human reproductive cloning should remain, as it is currently, illegal, the technique of cloning for the purpose of harvesting stem cells was morally acceptable and should be brought within the terms of the Human Fertilization and Embryology Act (1990). This Act permits the creation of embryos for research into infertility, stipulating that they should be destroyed after 14 days, which is the point at which the embryo would normally have implanted in the womb of the mother. The main ethical issue that arises in this technique is that the embryo is used for purposes other than reproduction, and is subsequently destroyed. If a life begins when fertilization takes place, then life is being destroyed for the sake of organ and tissue growth. A secondary issue is that the self-replication involved in cell nuclear transfer requires the availability of unfertilized eggs. If the person needing the organ or tissues is a woman she may be able to provide her own eggs, which would have to be removed surgically. If she is unable to provide her own eggs, or if the person is a man, the eggs would have to be donated, and there is already a general shortage of eggs for donation to women who are seeking in vitro fertilization anyway.

The fact that embryos are regarded by law as disposable items for 14 days does not mean that it is right that they are so regarded, and again, it is worth noting that if we were able to come up with a way of growing our own tissue without having to create embryos I am sure we would prefer to use such a method. Weiss thinks that eventually it may be possible.

Organ transplantation is a matter of life or death, and therefore research aimed at improving treatments in this area has to be supported. But in each of the techniques for producing new tissue so far discussed, harm is involved. The practices can be and have been justified by consequentialist arguments of need, and by risk–benefit analyses, where the benefits unquestionably outweigh the risks. But imagine being able to produce new tissue for patients without such a cost. Weiss thinks it is possible that we may eventually be able to regenerate organs from somatic, not embryonic cells, which would be preferable. It is less unnatural than taking foreign organs. If the research goals for organ transplantation were, in addition to saving life by these means, to find methods which harmed no-one, and which were as natural as possible, more effort might go into improving autografting techniques from somatic cells. I submit that no other technique will stand the test of time, because all the others require drastic interventions either to the host, or to the recipient, or both.

Methods of research

When designing a research project, it is essential that the researcher is clear what his hypothesis is. Popper's contribution to method in scientific discovery is immensely important, since by doing his best to *disprove* his hypothesis, rather than to prove it, the researcher is protected from seeing the evidence for his hypothesis wherever he looks, whilst ignoring anything else (Popper, 1959). But even with this safeguard, the fact remains that the hypothesis as it is fashioned will reflect what is normative for the researcher, and will determine everything about the way the research is conducted and the results that are achieved. By its very nature, then, planned research cannot produce another penicillin. Such discoveries can happen serendipitously, but that requires the researcher to remain open to developments that are wholly outside his normal experience. By the same token, results from other medical traditions, however unexpected they may be, should not be dismissed simply because they do not seem rational by an individual researcher's own standards.

The discovery of penicillin was due to luck and hard work, but not planning

Steven Lehrer's book *Explorers of the Body* (1979) is the source for this story, which begins with the work of Sir Almroth Wright (Sir Almost Right, as his detractors called him). He was the professor of pathology at the Army Medical School at Netley on Southampton Water in 1892. Very soon after his appointment there he produced a typhoid vaccine from killed typhoid bacillae. The vaccine attracted attention and interest because it was badly needed: many died from typhoid in England, and soldiers sent to hot climates in parts of the Empire were particularly susceptible. Encouraging early clinical trials led Wright to try to convince the Army authorities to vaccinate all the soldiers (numbering 320 000) going to the Boer War. The authorities remained dubious of the vaccine's efficacy, not least because Wright had broken with the Pasteur tradition by using killed vaccines. In the end only 16 000 soldiers were vaccinated. This could, in scientific terms, have been a perfect controlled trial, but the follow-up was somewhat messy. Apparently, for example, one medical orderly documented every man who contracted typhoid disease as having been vaccinated, believing that the fact they had the disease proved as much.

Wright was encouraged by such results as there were; others, however, remained sceptical. The continuing doubt in his findings culminated in Wright furiously resigning his post in the Army Medical School. Securing another professorship in pathology at St Mary's Hospital, Paddington, Wright continued to promote his vaccine. He won the favour of Lord Haldane, the Secretary of State for War, who said that the soldiers must be inoculated. The army establishment, however, remained unconvinced. Haldane said that Wright would have to become a 'public figure' in order for his work to be recognized by the establishment; accordingly, he had him knighted. Wright won the argument over the typhoid vaccine, and on account of his resolution in this matter his reputation grew, together with his confidence in the theory of immunity which he developed on the basis of these early successes. This theory, which he dubbed the opsonin theory, was a hybrid of two rival theories of immunity: the first being that factors in the blood fought off germs, and that vaccination produced these factors; the second, borrowed from another researcher called Metchnikoff, that cells will defend an organism against intruders. Metchnikoff called this action of the cells phagocytosis. Wright argued that the factors produced by vaccination in the circulating blood facilitated phagocytosis, thus far pre-empting modern theories of collaboration between antibodies and phagocytes. However, Wright further argued that the blood factors worked by making the germs more appetizing for the phagocytes. Wright coined the term opsonin from the Greek *opsono*, meaning, 'I prepare food for'.

Wright distilled his discoveries into an essential phrase: 'mobilize the immunological garrison'. This belief was partnered with the view that 'drugs are a delusion', because they could only repress symptoms, not provide a cure. This attitude pervaded the inoculation department at St Mary's Hospital when, in 1928, Alexander Fleming, a staff biologist, noted some strange behaviour in bacteria growing on a dish contaminated by mould.

In 1914, Fleming had conducted experiments as part of the War effort showing that antiseptic lotions applied to wounds did no good. They killed off the phagocytes, thus giving the germs the upper hand. Fleming became convinced that microbes, once in the body, could not be attacked. This belief seemed to be supported by other experiments conducted in 1922 in which he identified a substance called lysozyme.

The timing of the 1928 experiments was unbelievably lucky. When they were repeated, much later, it was found that the destructive effect of the mould on bacteria could not be produced at temperatures below 68 or above 90 degrees Fahrenheit. When Fleming performed his experiment there had been a heatwave followed by nine days of cold, when the temperature rose above 68 degrees only twice. Not only did Fleming's plate become contaminated with the one mould out of thousands that makes penicillin, it also happened when the ambient temperature was just right. A third piece of luck was observed by Dr Ernst Chaim in 1971. Fleming had thought he was looking at the effect that is the basis of penicillin's action against animal infections. In fact he was observing a special penicillin effect, seen in only a few bacterial species at just the right age and state of development.

But Fleming was too sceptical to believe he had found the long-sought-after drug capable of curing bacterial infection. His own war work and Wright's philosophy that 'drugs are a delusion' weighed too heavily against the significance of his findings. His simple, factual paper, with the crucial observation that the mould did not harm animals or humans, which later won him the Nobel Prize in medicine, went unnoticed by both fellow scientists and by pharmaceutical companies at the time. He was, by all accounts, very bad at communicating. Added to which, he was Wright's protégé and this made him unpopular with other bacteriologists at St Mary's, who by this time hated Wright in general because he was a despotic head of department, but in particular because he had put his own name to a paper which described work done by another (J.B. Freeman). The medical community outside St Mary's was hostile to Wright and his arrogance.

In his Nobel Prize speech Fleming justified himself thus:

My only merit is that I did not neglect the observation, and that I pursued it as a bacteriologist. The first practical use was to differentiate between different bacteria. We tried to concentrate penicillin but found, as others did later, that it was easily destroyed, and so, to all intents and purposes, we failed. Had I been an active clinician

I would doubtless have used it more extensively. (Lehrer, 1979, p. 307)

Privately he sounded more bitter:

I would have produced penicillin in 1929 if I had had the luck to have had a tame refugee chemist at my right hand. I had to stop where I did. (Lehrer, 1979, p. 307)

So Fleming had no chemist to help him. Wright, who believed chemists had not enough of the humanist in them to make them suitable colleagues in the pathology department, would not have them on his staff. The story of Fleming's two assistants, Craddock and Ridley, who were bacteriologists and therefore had to read up on chemistry as they went, is a tribute to the capacity to keep going in the most inauspicious circumstances. They gave up just one hurdle short of victory, though they were not to know that, having managed, in the most frightful conditions, to isolate the active residue of penicillin. Craddock later said:

We could not know at the time we had only one more hurdle to cross. We had been so often discouraged. We thought we had got the Thing. We put it into the refrigerator only to find, after a week, that it had begun to vanish. Had an experienced chemist come on the scene I think we could have got across that last hurdle. Then we could have published our results. But the expert did not materialise. (Lehrer, 1979, p. 311)

In 1929, just six months after Fleming had had his first glimpse of the activity of penicillin on a plate, the attempts to isolate the substance he had found came to an end. Ridley had boils and went on a cruise for his health. Craddock had just been married and secured a better position at the Wellcome Research Laboratories. Fleming made no immediate effort to find anyone to continue the work. He was so influenced by Wright's philosophy, which also included the view that animals were not appropriate models for humans, that he did not inject the extract into bacterially infected mice, an obvious next step to today's scientific mind.

In 1931 Raistrick, a chemist, took the experiments further but was, like Fleming, still unaware of the therapeutic implications of penicillin. He was able to make the substance dissolve in ether, which Craddock and Ridley had been unable to do. However, when he found that it disappeared along with the ether when the ether was evaporated to extract the penicillin, he gave up and turned his mind to other experiments. Like Fleming, he lost his assistants. Like Fleming, he did not replace them because he did not appreciate how important the work was.

Lewis Holt picked up the pieces where Raistrick left off, but he was only shown Raistrick's assistants' work, not that of Craddock and Ridley. Lewis found a way of preserving the penicillin whilst evaporating the ether but he was thwarted by penicillin's instability and gave up. Fleming did not encourage him to continue trying. Meanwhile, Dr C.G. Paine in 1931 employed penicillin therapeutically with dramatic results; he however began to find difficulty producing more penicillin in that some was highly active and some not at all active. He too gave up, later saying that he was transferred to a different line of work which, together with the failure to produce more penicillin, made him feel it was the right decision at the time. His experiments were never published in scientific journals.

Although four articles were written on penicillin between 1928 and 1935, no one believed a substance produced in a petri dish could treat animal infection. German chemists at the soon-to-be notorious I.G. Farben Industrie (which later produced Zyklon B gas), were working during the 1930s on finding a more penetrative and hence more effective dye. One such new dye was called Prontosil. A Dr Domagh, Director of research at the German Bayer company, a subsidiary of Farben, tested Prontosil as part of a mass screening programme to detect chemicals that might be effective in treating infections. He was using animals for experimental purposes. He had already discovered that some chemicals, which showed no activity in test tubes, were active in animals. Prontosil showed dramatic effects in animals, and then in humans, the first of whom to be given the substance was Domagh's daughter, who was dying of septicaemia caused by pricking herself with a knitting needle. She, and 1500 treated patients after her, survived and recovered.

There followed a three year hiatus. Domagh was arranging iron-clad patents. But research on Prontosil in France pre-empted him. The French researchers isolated sulfanilamide as the active molecule of the two into which Prontosil split when it entered the body. Because of earlier, though abandoned, experiments with this substance, it was not possible to patent it. Colebrooke at St Mary's, experimenting on all subjects (having decided it would be unethical to treat only half of them, though this would have been more rigorous scientifically), showed remarkable results.

However, sulfanilamide was active against some bacteria but not others. Medical research continued to look for more effective anti-bacterial compounds, and the interest was now keen, for the prejudice had finally broken down against systemic antibacterial therapy.

Howard Walter Florey from Adelaide in South Australia was the one who finally brought the project to a successful *finale*. When he was appointed to the Chair of Pathology at Oxford he determined to create what we would now call a multi-disciplinary department, with integrated bacteriology, chemical pathology and biochemistry. Funds were very short; Oxford University and the Medical Research Council refused support, and the bright stars Florey had attracted to his department were threatening to leave. The Rockefeller Foundation stepped in and it was Florey's department, free from prejudice and with different disciplines playing their rightful parts, which succeeded in producing penicillin. On Saturday May 25th 1940, experiments in mice were totally successful.

By 1943 American and British army doctors were administering penicillin,

dramatically increasing the survival of soldiers suffering from wound infections. After the War, the availability of penicillin completely changed the
course of bacterial diseases which had hitherto been killers.

Of course, penicillin is not the holy grail it appeared to be when its
characteristics were finally recognized and put to use. Its extensive use not
only produces (albeit minimally harmful and still outweighed by the benefits)
side effects in the individual, it also gives rise to problems of resistance
generally. The purpose of telling the story, however, is not to celebrate the
drug's discovery as an unqualified success, but rather to consider the implications of how it was discovered. It was a case not so much of 'seeing is
believing' as of needing to believe in order to see, or at least to be open to the
possibility of believing before being able to see. Once the belief was there, and
the evidence began to support it, energy and resources began to be made
available for further research and exploration.

Alternative and complementary therapy research needs open minds

Some publications about trials in homeopathy show an uncanny resemblance
to the penicillin story. Stacey (1991) says it is a failure of Western scientific
models to understand anything of alternative medicine, not just individual
myopia, that gives rise to the refusal to accept that alternative medicine
works.

For some time now alternative approaches to medicine have become
increasingly popular, and numerous traditional methods are reappearing:
'All these ways of healing have burgeoned forth, like a stream re-appearing
from underground in limestone country, a stream which had been eclipsed
but was not eliminated' (Stacey, 1991). Brewin (1993), in a critical article,
puts the popularity down to a series of factors. First, patients desire more
time and attention from doctors, including more sympathetic understanding
and, in some cases, hope. Then, they desire to be given causes and explanations. In the case of serious illness, the desire to try anything and everything is
very strong, often accompanied with a desire to feel in control of the
situation, instead of accepting circumstances and facing the unknown. Finally, alternative, or fringe as Brewin calls it, medicine appeals to that side of our
nature which prefers magic to logic, which he thinks is evidence of a basic
instinct we all have that is trying to find other outlets since the decline of
religious affiliation. He observes that fringe medicine is not logical, since it
conducts very little testing of remedies, very little self-criticism or learning
from mistakes, and is usually based on beliefs without adequate supporting
evidence. He identifies fringe medicine's use of 'bad magic' in its assumption
that human life was healthier when it was more natural and less civilized,
even though, as he points out, today we generally enjoy a safer life, a better
quality of life, and a longer life than our ancestors (at any rate in the West).

Fringe medicine suffers from the belief that a healthy mind protects us from all ills, and it also takes the view that mainstream medicine has failed if it has not cured. In fairness, Brewin observes that mainstream medicine is as prone to believing in magic as fringe medicine is, so that claims by the World Health Organization to bring about 'health for all by the year 2000' seem as far fetched as the claim in the *Oxford Handbook of Complementary Medicine* that 'homeopathy can be successful in all diseases'. He runs through a series of propositions that mainstream medicine has failed to take account of in the past, leading to some really useless or downright harmful treatments being perpetuated in the firm belief that they work. He observes, for example, that if treatment A has better results than treatment B, then it may be that treatment A is useless and treatment B is harmful; also, if an assortment of widely different treatments all give broadly the same result, they may all be useless. The only way that mainstream medicine is to rid itself of its tendency to believe in magic is by carefully controlled comparison trials, starting with pilot trials. Brewin wonders why nobody thought of comparative trials before now. He throws down the gauntlet to fringe medicine to subject itself to just such comparisons; he asks, for example, why the Bristol Cancer Help Centre did not subject its very exacting special diet to a comparison trial, whereby all the participants received the same treatment from the Centre, but the treatment group received the special diet and the control group received an ordinary well-balanced diet. Would it be the case, though, that had such a trial taken place and the conclusion been that the diet did work, that that conclusion would have been discounted by those who start with an assumption such as that food is not medicine? This is the kind of obstacle that those who champion evidence-based medicine are up against.

Trials in homeopathy

One area of fringe or alternative medicine that has taken the gauntlet of comparison trials is homeopathy, not least because of all the varieties of alternative treatment this is the most amenable to such trials. In 1994, D. Reilly and others published a paper in the *Lancet* giving the results of a trial which sought to reproduce the evidence of two previous trials that homeopathy differs from placebo. The test model was homeopathic immunotherapy. The summary stated:

Twenty-eight patients with allergic asthma, most of them sensitive to house-dust mite, were randomly allocated to receive either oral homeopathic immunotherapy to their principal allergen or identical placebo. The test treatments were given as a complement to the unaltered conventional care. A daily visual analogue scale of overall symptom intensity was the outcome measure. A difference in visual analogue score in favour of homeopathic immunotherapy appeared within one week of starting treatment and persisted for up to eight weeks ($p = 0.003$). There were similar trends in respiratory function and bronchial reactivity tests.

A meta-analysis of all three trials strengthened the evidence that homeopathy does more than placebo ($p = 0.0004$). Is the reproducibility of evidence in favour of homeopathy proof of its activity or proof of the clinical trial's capacity to produce false-positive results? (Reilly et al., 1994).

In 1997 *The Lancet* published a meta-analysis on homeopathic trials together with two unfavourable commentaries (Langman, 1997; Linde et al., 1997; Vandenbroucke, 1997). Interestingly, the authors of both commentaries find themselves unable to believe the results, not because the evidence is unconvincing, but because they simply cannot believe that a treatment which is the result of a series of dilutions, such that there are no molecules left at all of the original substance, can work. Jan P. Vandenbroucke states: 'Bayesian investigators will remain unimpressed by the results of homeopathy trials; when there is no convincing theory underlying a trial, the results will remain uninterpretable'. He acknowledges that this has implications for the status of evidence for trials in allopathic medicine, as Reilly anticipated. Vandenbroucke writes: 'It might be impossible to identify false-positive findings in trials of allopathic medicines, because our belief in the proposed mechanisms could blind us to the possibility that the trial results are wrong' (Vandenbroucke, 1997). The other commentator concludes:

Their [the authors of the meta-analysis] careful analyses expose sources of bias, but there is enough in the study to give sound reasoning for asking for good controlled trials. However, the scientist must question whether the diversion of significant resources to support these trials can be justified when a rational basis for choice of homeopathy, or any particular modality of it, is lacking. (Langman, 1997)

The failure of these two commentators to accept evidence, or to agree that if this evidence is not sound enough that further research is justified, is based upon their inability to believe that homeopathy can work. Although such a failure of belief is understandable (how can something work that is not there?), these commentators demonstrate the same sort of lack of logic that Brewin so decried in his earlier article. It resonates with the prejudices of the staff biologists in Sir Almroth Wright's department at St Mary's, Paddington. It was their firm belief that microbes, once in the body, could not be attacked, and that nothing that was prepared in a petri dish could treat animal infection, that prevented Fleming from seeing what he was looking at, as it were.

Reilly writes:

The usual response to the possibility that homeopathic treatments are effective is to call for a mechanism of action – asking 'how?' before asking 'if?' is a bad basis for good science when dealing empirically with things that may as yet evade explanation. (Reilly et al., 1994).

He then goes on to speculate as to how it is that homeopathy works, as follows:

Opposite action at low dose – a poison becoming an aid – is not unfamiliar in conventional science and is the subject of much debate... For today's science, however, the main barrier to acceptance of homeopathy is the issue of serially vibrated dilutions that lack any molecules at all of the original substance. Can water or alcohol of fixed biochemical composition encode differing biological information? Using current metaphors, does the chaos-inducing vibration, central to the production of a homeopathic dilution, encourage biophysically different fractal-like patterns of the diluent, critically dependent upon the starting conditions? Theoretical physicists seem more at ease with such ideas than pharmacologists, considering the possibilities of isotopic stereodiversity, clathrates, or resonance and coherence within water as possible modes of transmission, while other workers are exploring the idea of electromagnetic changes. Nuclear magnetic resonance changes in homeopathic dilutions have been reported and, if reproducible, may be offering us a glimpse of a future territory.

Dissemination of the results of research

Chapter Two discussed the numerous problems which arise from trying to disseminate the results of research, despite the importance of doing so. The cases discussed in this section illustrate some of the problems. In particular, they demonstrate the influence of the motives of the researchers in their choice of research question and inevitably in the results they generate. These results can be useless or even seriously misleading to those who do not share the views of the researchers, which is often the position of the patients whom the research was supposed to help.

Results of research into futile treatment depend on what is understood by 'futile'

Harper (1998) wrote about the issue of research into futile treatment. His study is fascinating because of the light it sheds upon the relationship between the intentions and beliefs of the researcher, the research question, the method used in the research, and the answer gained. He agreed that it was not good that doctors should offer experimental treatments more than a very few times to their patients at the end of their lives, on the shaky grounds that it might help and nothing else at this stage has. Clearly, any treatment that might be thought to help should be subjected to proper and controlled testing to see whether the hunch of the doctor was right or not. But the research question that is put to such a treatment is all important, not only for the design and conduct of the trial but also for the use to which the trial data can then be put once they have been generated. William Harper cites a number of trials on treatments routinely given in intensive care, which concluded that such treatments were futile. Judgements of medical futility are, he argues, value laden and differ amongst medical professionals even when there is agreement on the facts of the case. For example, he asks, is the administering of cardio-pulmonary resuscitation (CPR), which offers a child only three more days of life, still dependent upon intensive care, futile or not? In his paper, Harper cites a study by Lantos, which concluded that CPR should not be offered to low-birth-weight babies routinely because it was in many cases futile; the outcome measurement in Lantos' trial was survival to hospital discharge. As Harper points out, such a question will be felt to be more-or-less relevant depending on the individual concerned. Some will feel that it is appropriate whilst others might feel that even a few days of life are better than none, and worth the treatment. Harper's concern is not whether those who would choose to have the extra time are wrong in their views, but rather that Lantos' study could not provide them with information they would want to know in order to decide whether to allow CPR for their child or not, unless they studied his method. Lantos' study would be helpful only to those who, effectively, agree with his initial premise: that treatment which does not give survival to hospital discharge is futile.

Results of pharmaceutical company research are always commercially favourable

A similar issue arises within pharmaceutical company research, when the clear aim of a company is to show that its drugs successfully treat certain conditions. A trial can be designed to do this, providing the question is right. Toine Pieters showed that the three pharmaceutical companies which had most heavily invested in interferon in the 1970s managed, by dint of much 'fishing', to find the right answers to the use of the drug (namely, within a multitreatment framework). As Pieters put it:

They tried different combinations and different routes and durations of administration. In doing so, they ultimately tinkered towards success in terms of establishing new therapeutic drug practices for interferon and actively working on the treatment's effectiveness... In positioning interferon as a 'helpful neighbour', compatible with and supportive of existing treatment practices, the pharmaceutical companies succeeded in having interferon relatively quickly absorbed into the medical infrastructure. (Pieters, 1998)

In his discussion of research into futile treatment, Harper identifies three reasons why research should not be narrowly focused. First, the decision about whether or not to let a patient die is one over which informed and well-intentioned people form different moral judgements. Moreover, it is a deeply personal decision, which needs adequate information, and the research done so far does not offer such information. If the gathering and dissemination of information is limited to the personal concerns and beliefs of the researcher, this imposes his judgement as to when a life is worth living on to those who use the results of his research. In such cases as these, the pressure to use evidence-based medicine can be positively counter to patients' interests. A second reason for not narrowly defining research goals is that a researcher with unpopular value judgements may be frozen out of funding. The spate of trials into futile treatment in intensive care in the UK was a response to the Government's concern about the cost of such treatment in the state-funded health service. If the sponsors of research want a particular answer to a question, it may well be a matter of simply making sure that the question is right, then the desired answer may be gained. The third reason Harper identifies is that medicine is a social enterprise, and research should be aimed at meeting public needs, not the wishes of individuals.

Results should ultimately meet public need

Research should not be narrowly focused because medicine is a social enterprise, existing at the service of the public. Hence, allowing the personal values of researchers to 'choke off' (Harper, 1998) the information the public needs to make responsible decisions about its own health care is inappropriate. This third reason has given the spur to the considerable efforts being made to include consumer groups in the initiation and design of research protocols. Chalmers (1995), in particular, has argued that including such groups makes a big difference to the research questions being asked. He cites, as an example of the usefulness of consumer perspective, the trial on the efficacy of intensive monitoring of fetuses during labour. The trial showed that this monitoring decreased the chances of a baby having seizures. The difference the monitoring made was statistically significant, but, to women going through labour, the encumbrance of being connected to fetal monitoring equipment during labour was not worth the potential benefit – for the difference in the number of babies with seizures dropped from 998 in one thousand to 996. This study is a good example of MacRae's point that statistics are simply mathematics, but the clinically relevant difference a treatment makes is a value judgement which should not be made by a statistician, but by those whose interests are affected by the outcome.

Summary and concluding remarks

This chapter has considered the practical implications of the goal-based approach to moral thinking under three headings: the goals of research; the design of research; and the dissemination of the results of research, following the pattern of the discussion in Chapter Two. Specific examples of questions and problems in these three areas were looked at. Under goals of research organ transplantation was considered. The different sorts of investigations and treatments that have been, and are being, developed for this medical need were looked at. At each stage, the treatments involve actions which involve some risk of harm. The assumption that this had to be so was challenged, wondering whether Weiss' view that it should be possible to grow autografts without creating human embryos could not be realized.

The section on methods in research described the story of the discovery of penicillin, which had to wait upon the attitudes and beliefs of the clinicians of the time before its properties were realized. Similar reactions to research into complementary medicine were then described. The research and the treatments may in fact be unsuccessful, but mere prejudice will not prove that any more than it will recognize success.

Finally, in discussing the dissemination of results of research, research into so-called futile treatments, pharmaceutical company research, and research into fetal monitoring during labour were looked at. In all three cases, the intentions of the researchers or the ones commissioning the research were out of line with those of the people who would make use of the results of the research.

All these examples of issues which arise in the context of goal-based thinking raise serious questions about how research goals are set and met. The goals of research arise out of the motives of researchers or their sponsors. The motivation for undertaking research is varied: there may be simple curiosity about how something works or whether it is possible to achieve something, or there may be a clear recognition of a medical need and potential way of meeting it; there may be commercial motivations, or selfish ones. This chapter suggested that the goals of research are lent moral validity by their being placed within a wider goal of complete cures with no side effects. In serving these goals, there need be no fundamental assumptions about what will and what will not work. There certainly need not be the belief that there are no medical benefits without associated harms, even if the evidence appears that there is no gain without pain. Setting aside assumptions of this sort opens the possibility of bold, even quantum leaps in our knowledge and understanding of medical care. It also facilitates the work of those who seek to educate the medical profession into using evidence-based medicine. The intuition and experience which it was argued were an essential part of a good doctor's approach to his patients should, therefore, always be subject to the possibility of change.

7

Case studies of duty-based issues

Introduction

Chapter Three sought to establish the validity of the duty-based perspective in moral thinking by showing some of its foundations, namely the tradition of natural law ethics, and the Kantian categorical imperative. It suggested that the practical implication for the ethics of research on humans of the duty-based moral perspective is that, by virtue of their function, the doctor/researchers have a duty to care for each of their patient/participants, which they exercise by acting only in their best interests. This duty has no contingent justification. It is absolute, inherent in the function of the doctor. Hence, a research project might be aiming at a goal which is good, and it might have the agreement of the research participants who are to help achieve the goal, but it still needs to be justified according to duty-based criteria, namely that it is in the patients' best interests that they participate.

The issues that arise in the context of duty-based morality in research do so because of clashes with competing goal- and right-based moral claims. The examples investigated in this chapter will show how this happens. Clashes with goal-based morality happen frequently in therapeutic research with the question of whether or not there should be a placebo control with which to compare the experimental treatment. Goal-based morality, expressed as scientific rigour, demands that new treatments are compared with placebo unless there are compelling reasons to the contrary. Duty-based morality, expressed as a patient's best interest, demands that no placebo arm be included if a standard treatment is available. Both points of view are based on ethical thinking but they do not accord with each other.

In some trials, placebos were omitted on ethical grounds. This is illogical because studies destined to produce unreliable results should themselves be considered unethical. (Tramer *et al.*, 1998).

This statement demonstrates a muddle between two competing ethical principles. One principle is that it is wrong to harm research subjects by offering a placebo when an active treatment is available (duty-based); the other is that it is wrong to conduct research which produces uninterpretable results, which the omission of a placebo arm can do (goal-based). Both principles are valid, but the two do not necessarily work together. It is not, therefore, illogical to say that placebo controlled trials needed for scientific purposes are nevertheless unethical, they are just unethical for different reasons from scientific ones. Resolution of the dilemma, if it is possible, will only happen if the two needs are clearly seen, together with the extent of their claim on our moral attention. Hence, the arguments for and against the use of placebo will be considered in some depth, using as examples trials of folic acid in pregnancy, trials of treatments of peptic ulcer disease, and trials of ondansetron for post-operative nausea and vomiting.

In non-therapeutic research the clash between goal-based scientific concerns and duty-based concerns for adequate care of individuals can arise even more acutely. By way of demonstration a trial which involved placing babies in chambers with reduced oxygen to investigate a possible cause of sudden infant death syndrome will be considered.

The clash between duty-based and right-based moral perspectives shows itself when potential research subjects are willing to participate in research, so fulfilling the right-based requirement to consult those most affected by the action, but who, according to a duty-based view, should not have been asked in the first place, or whose request to participate should have been refused, because of the risks involved. The example considered to illustrate this difficulty is non-therapeutic research on competent subjects, namely, Phase I, healthy volunteer pharmaceutical trials, when drugs are given for the first time to human beings. Here, the research subjects' consent is carefully sought before they are enrolled. The adequacy of the consent procedure is not in question here, so it is a good example to use to demonstrate the tension that can genuinely arise between duty-based and right-based morality.

Therapeutic research

Duty to care versus scientific goals: placebo controls in therapeutic research

As discussed in Chapter Three, the researcher conducting therapeutic research needs to be in strong equipoise for duty-based morality to be honoured. This means her duty to care for each of her patients must be active: she must act in her patients' best interests, and so she must be entirely happy that the treatment that each of her patients receives in the trial is the best as far as she knows. It follows that each of the arms of a trial to which her patient may be allocated must be as good as the others, as far as she can tell. A placebo arm, where no treatment is on offer, can only ethically (in the duty-based sense) be included if no 'proven, available treatment' exists (World Medical Association, 1996). If a treatment did exist, then the doctor is morally obliged to offer it. Not to do so would be equivalent to offering her patient, who presents with an illness in ordinary circumstances, a pink pill instead of a proper drug, when the proper drug is available. In some cases, the novel and untested treatment is so likely to be of some use that it is unethical to deny it to anyone. This was the position of Colebrook with penicillin. In other cases, patients may have such life-threatening conditions that denying them treatment would be unacceptable.

The goal-based argument for including placebo arms except in unavoidable cases, such as where the patients' condition is life threatening, is that without them most trial results are uninterpretable. It is not worth conducting randomized controlled trials of new treatments if there cannot be a placebo arm, because the researcher can never otherwise know the extent to which a new treatment is genuinely causal of an improvement in a condition, or whether the improvement would have happened without any active intervention. Active drug comparators cannot provide this information. In any case they themselves may never have been proved against placebo. If there is more than one possible active comparator, there is no reliable way of establishing which of them, and at which dose, can be the gold standard comparator for the treatment being tested.

Trials of folic acid in pregnancy

The example of the trials into folic acid in pregnancy illustrate the puzzle of whether or not to use placebo controls (Scott et al., 1994). If, in the early days of pregnancy, the neural plate of the fetus does not close to form the neural tube which encompasses the spine and the brain, either spina bifida results, if the spine is not properly enclosed, or anencephaly, if the brain is not properly enclosed. It was thought that if the mother took folic acid she could help prevent the tragedy of neural tube defects. A research project was proposed to test folic acid against placebo to see if the hypothesis was correct. But the research ethics committee which had to give the study its approval decided that it was unethical to deny folic acid to anyone, because there were many indications that folic acid did indeed make a considerable difference to the development of the fetus. In the event, the control group consisted of those mothers not in the trial. Interpretation of the results was so difficult that another, placebo controlled, trial was set up and conducted by the Medical Research Council (MRC) to resolve the question. That trial found that if mothers took 4 mg per day of folic acid the chances of neural tube defects reduced by three quarters.

It could be argued, from a duty-based perspective, that the fears of the earlier research ethics committee were realized, for in the MRC trial the women randomized to the placebo arm were denied treatment which was found to be extremely effective. From a goal-based perspective, however, the MRC research was justified by its result, because it demonstrated that folic acid did indeed make a difference, something the earlier, non-randomized trial had not been able to demonstrate. All the research ethics committee had done, on this argument, was to delay the truth being discovered, and hence to expose numerous women, more than the number who were allocated placebo in the MRC trial, to the risk of pregnancy without folic acid. Moreover, the value of folic acid is found only if it is taken around the time of conception and then in the early days of pregnancy (because neural tube defects occur early). Since numerous pregnancies are not planned, or, if they are planned, conception does not take place as soon as contraception is withdrawn, it is difficult to persuade women of child-bearing potential to take folic acid on a semi-permanent basis, just in case they fall pregnant. The results of the research needed to be absolutely certain for the advice to take folic acid to be worth the effort. The goal-based justification for the placebo controlled trials is cast iron. But the duty-based concern is also genuine. There will have been women whose babies were born with spina bifida or anencephaly, whose researching clinicians will have been aware of a way, unsubstantiated but likely to be effective, of lessening the risk of that happening, but who denied them the treatment. The researcher in a person might be able to turn a blind eye to the individual woman's plight, in the certainty of the importance of the research for millions of (other) women in the future. The doctor in the same person might not be capable of such scientific *sang froid*, unless he was convinced that folic acid might not do any good at all. The case demonstrates the conflict.

Trials for treatments of peptic ulcer disease

The debate between those who favour placebo controlled trials and those who do not is a debate between goal-based thinkers who would always use a placebo unless there were compelling reasons not to, and duty-based thinkers who would only use a placebo if there was no alternative. Writing in favour of the use of placebo controls for trials into treatments of peptic ulcer disease, Ciociola and others (1996) provide some powerful arguments on the goal-based side. There are plenty of 'proven, available' treatments for peptic ulcer disease. Hence, from a duty-based perspective, no trial of new treatments should have placebo comparators, because to deny people with the disease a treatment which was available would be to act against their best interests. But, argues Ciociola, placebo therapy is effective in 48% to 58% of cases of peptic ulcer disease. What that means is that giving dummy substances to people with peptic ulcers has resulted in about half of them getting better. In a trial without a placebo arm, it will not be possible to know if the effects that are seen from the treatments given in the trial are from the content of the pills, or just from the act of taking the pills. It is necessary, then, to have a placebo arm to establish the baseline remission rate of the disease. Also, the safety data for the new chemical entity being researched will not be adequate until the research has taken place. It is ethical, argues Ciociola, to offer the drug with its unknown side effects to as few patients as possible until more is known. Placebo controlled trials require far fewer participants than active comparator trials. Type I and Type II errors are inversely proportional to the number of participants needed in the trial.

As explained in Chapter Two, a Type I, or Alpha error, is the probability of falsely rejecting the null hypothesis, which means that the treatments appear to be different, but in fact they are the same. For a trial to be considered valid, it must have a p or probability value of less than 5%. A Type II, or Beta error, is the probability of failing to reject the null hypothesis when in fact there is a difference between the two treatments. This is regarded as less serious than a Type I error, and hence the probability is allowed to be greater, 20%, or to put it another way, a probability of rejecting the null hypothesis when the null hypothesis is false of 80%.

In a theoretical example, Ciociola shows that a placebo controlled study needs only 28 patients in each of the active and placebo arms, or on a 2:1 ratio, which is statistically acceptable, 42 patients in the active arm and 21 in the placebo arm, for the study to avoid both Alpha and Beta errors. If the study were to be conducted as an active drug comparator study, with no placebo arm, 408 patients would be needed in each arm to avoid Alpha and Beta errors.

Ciociola concludes that placebo controlled trials should be conducted for new peptic ulcer treatments, as long as high-risk patients are eliminated and supplemental antacids are available to the placebo arm. We can appreciate that from his perspective, which recognizes the goal-based need for the research to be done scientifically, this is the most ethical approach. But it could equally well be argued, from a duty-based perspective, that it is worse to deny treatment to patients than it is to conduct scientifically valid studies; that if it is wrong to give an untested treatment whose safety data is not adequate to many people, then it is equally wrong to give it even to one person. If a project needs 816 rather than 56 or 63 patients to be valid then it should recruit that number, rather than compromise duty-based principles.

Scientific arguments against the use of placebo

The problem in seeking to ensure that ethical research is conducted is that the goal-based and duty-based perspectives often do not speak in a mutually meaningful language to each other in order to find a resolution when they clash. Goal-based morality uses the language of science; duty-based morality uses the language of doctors' duties. Freedman's analysis of the arguments for placebo controlled trials (Freedman et al., 1997a, b) may be useful in this respect. He concludes that placebo arms are justified in only four circumstances, so taking the duty-based line that reasons have to be found for using placebo controls rather than for not using them. But many of his arguments are scientific. Thus, he meets goal-based thinkers on their own territory. He thinks that the belief that having a placebo arm provides a reliable baseline against which to test whether a new treatment works is too simplistic. It presumes the existence of two sets of causes for a drug's effectiveness – psychological and biological – that act independently, so that by subtracting one of these sets from the group's results, the other remains (as in Ciociola's justification for a placebo arm to factor out the placebo, or psychological, effect). This notion ignores the possible synergistic actions of the two causes. For example, the psychological expectation of benefit might be reinforced by a subject's perception of improvement caused by biological factors. In this model, the placebo effect of active drugs would be greater than the placebo effect of placebos.

The placebo effect is well-documented, says Freedman. Different coloured placebos, for example, have had different effects on those who take them. What sort of placebo should be used for a baseline? He suggests that a trial of a drug which suppresses the appetite which compares the (blue) active drug with an identical placebo might show the active drug to be superior. But suppose the active and placebo tablets had been red? It may be that in a red tablet the placebo effect would be potentiated and the difference between the drug and the placebo eliminated or rendered non-significant. Freedman cites Philip's paradox: that placebo controlled trials are only successful when they reveal no advantage for the experimental intervention over placebo; that is, positive results of placebo controlled trials are uninterpretable because the more effective an experimental treatment is, the more likely it is to become unblinded (obvious to all concerned that it is the active drug) during the study, rendering it impossible to state whether the observed advantage of the experimental arm is due to its inherent activity or to the expectancy effect it has generated.

The FDA's arguments for requiring placebo

The United States' Food and Drug Administration (FDA), which is responsible for licensing all new drugs for marketing in the US, has stated that it will require placebo controlled trials to demonstrate a new drug's efficacy in all but trials of treatments for life-threatening conditions. This is significant for medicines research around the world, for all pharmaceutical companies wish to sell their drugs in the lucrative United States market. Hence, the stipulations of the FDA set the international standard for medicines research. The FDA requires placebo controlled trials to be the norm. The 1962 amendments to the Food and Drug Act (Food, Drug and Cosmetic Act, 1938) expanded the FDA's role to include an evaluation of a drug's effectiveness by requiring 'substantial evidence that the drug will have the effect it purports'. 'Substantial evidence' is defined in the Act as follows:

Adequate and well-controlled investigations, including clinical investigations, by experts qualified by scientific training and experience to evaluate the effectiveness of the drug involved, on the basis of which it could fairly and responsibly be concluded by such experts that the drug will have the effect it purports or is represented to have under the conditions of use prescribed, recommended, or suggested in the labelling or proposed labelling thereof.

The way this requirement has been interpreted is that absolute effectiveness has to be demonstrated, that is, that a new drug is better than nothing; rather than relative effectiveness, that is, that a new drug is comparable to, or better than, the standard drugs already available. Many would agree that placebo controlled trials are justifiable if the standard treatments which would otherwise be the comparator have not themselves been proved against placebo, but even when standard treatments have been so proved, the FDA insists that the comparator for any new drug should still be placebo. Freedman responds passionately:

To understand effectiveness in this (absolute) way is absurd; by this measure, flinging a glass of water at a burning building is an effective fire-fighting strategy because it is better than nothing. The public knows that FDA represents a massive, expensive bureaucracy, needing to fulfil its role as a gatekeeper of new drugs. But how many health care professionals or lay members of the public are aware that because of its reliance on placebo controls, the normal operation of FDA may result in the licensure of a new drug inferior in every way to presently available treatment? And how many are aware that to fulfil this mandate, FDA will not licence new drugs unless the manufacturer runs trials that are contrary to numerous authoritative pronouncements on research ethics, both national and international? (Freedman et al., 1997b).

Robert Temple (1996) has been influential in maintaining the view within the FDA that the goal-based scientific arguments for placebo controlled trials are pre-eminent. Like others, he argues that active control trials (where the comparator is the standard available treatment rather than placebo) present insuperable statistical difficulties. Freedman disagrees, presenting an alternative trial design which aims to show active control equivalence. In this design, two treatments are compared, not to test if one is superior, but to test whether they are equivalent. The null hypothesis is that the treatments differ by more than some defined amount; the alternate hypothesis is that the two treatments differ by less than that defined amount. The hypotheses are thus a reversal of the hypotheses in placebo controlled trials. They can be designed around conventional values of Type I and Type II errors. The sample sizes of these studies fall between the large numbers needed for active control studies, and the small numbers needed for placebo controlled studies. Others have offered advice on ways to make these trials as reliable as possible (Jones et al.,

1996). However, it must be recognized that such trials are not as statistically rigorous as placebo controlled trials, and if the goal-based moralist is not inclined to give any concessions to the duty-based perspective (except to recognize extreme cases of risk), she is not going to give up her own trial design in favour of an inferior one. For even though Freedman uses scientific language, he makes allowances for the need for scientific rigour only after the duty-based demand to give patients treatment in their best interests has been satisfied. His arguments start from a duty-based perspective, whereas those of Temple and the FDA start with the goal-based need for rigorous science, making allowances for duty-based ethical demands to treat patients according to their best interests. Thus, the two approaches do not really meet in the middle, despite Freedman's attempts to make them do so.

Meta-analysis of trials of ondansetron

The trials of ondansetron are a practical demonstration of the difficulty as it is currently being faced by researchers and research ethics committees. Ondansetron is a treatment for postoperative nausea and vomiting. When ondansetron trials began to take place during the early 1990s, considerable concern was expressed over whether these trials should be placebo controlled or not, because of the existence of so many other treatments, none of which, however, had been established as best practice. As a consequence, of the many trials of ondansetron which took place, some of them were placebo controlled, some with and some without an active comparator arm, and some were active comparator only. Aspinall and Goodman (1995) were concerned not only that as many as 2620 patients were denied existing drugs in the trials they reviewed from the published literature, but also that trials which only showed that ondansetron was better than placebo provided clinicians with insufficient information as to whether or not to use ondansetron, since they were not thereby informed of other drugs to treat the same condition, nor of their relative efficacy against ondansetron.

Three years later, Tramer et al. (1998) were to use the trials in ondansetron to demonstrate that placebo controlled trials are essential. They chose studies of this drug because placebo controlled trials had been repeatedly questioned, and because they already had good estimates of ondansetron's anti-emetic efficacy and harm postoperatively, from a systematic review of the trials, against which to compare the active controlled trials.

A review of all the active controlled trials was conducted. Many different regimens of ondansetron had been compared with many different anti-emetic controls, demonstrating how much uncertainty there was about which regimen of ondansetron is the best and which active comparator should be the gold standard active control. Of the placebo controlled trials, whatever the dose of ondansetron used, ondansetron showed superiority over placebo. But of the placebo group, variations of nausea and vomiting ranged from 10% to 96% up to 48 hours postoperatively. The significance this result presented for the meaningful interpretation of results was that if some patients do not vomit postoperatively anyway, then prophylactic anti-emetic efficacy cannot be shown; if all patients vomit then it will be exaggerated.

Many of the trials showed no difference between ondansetron and the active comparator. This failure to show a difference does not necessarily mean equivalence, however, despite Freedman's claims. In an equivalence trial, Tramer argues, we need to know the extent of the placebo response, and that it does not vary. Otherwise, two active treatments showing the same result could simply mean that both are equally ineffective. One trial showed a remarkable result: ondansetron was equivalent to placebo but better than the active drug. This was evidence of internal insensitivity of the trial, and this was only detectable because there was a placebo arm.

The scattergram Tramer produced, which compared ondansetron with other drugs, suggested that ondansetron was no better than any of the other drugs, except possibly metoclopramide. However, because the optimal dose of metoclopramide is not known, it is not known if patients in the trial were just given too little of the drug for it to take effect. The absence of placebo in the active control trials meant that they could not inform as to the rates of nausea and vomiting without anti-emetic prophylaxis in these study populations, nor did they have an index of internal sensitivity. Hence, argues Tramer, their results cannot be interpreted. The conclusion of these authors was that placebo is justified in ondansetron trials because of the underlying variation in likelihood of nausea and vomiting and because of the lack of a gold standard comparator.

These two reasons are goal-based, however. From that perspective, they are justified, adequate reasons for including a placebo arm. But from a duty-based perspective, a placebo controlled trial of ondansetron means a group of patients will not receive treatment for postoperative nausea and vomiting when many commonly-used treatments exist. Many patients suffer from nausea and vomiting. From the duty-based perspective, perfectly good treatments are being denied to patients in the interests of science and society, as Aspinall and Goodman pointed out. The goal-based response to this might be to underline the fact that postoperative nausea and vomiting are not life-threatening conditions, and the importance of establishing the truth about the efficacy of treatments for the condition outweighs the discomfort that the patients may feel by being denied treatment. The duty-based moralist will not accept such a view, because it keeps the goal of the research in a superior position to the individual interests of the research participants. Indeed, the assertion that it is important to establish the truth about ondansetron gives support to the duty-based approach, for it means the condition which it is hoped to treat is one that *should* be treated. So, to emphasize the point, some patients in the trial are being denied treatment for a condition which should be treated, and which may not kill them but is horrible to experience, for the sake of science and society.

Concluding remarks

From the range of views identified above, we can see that to decide whether or not a trial should be placebo controlled rests on whether we tend to be more goal-based or more duty-based in our thinking. The goal-based approach is to conduct placebo controlled trials wherever possible, only avoiding them when there is likelihood of real harm. The assumption is that the placebo controlled trial is the better trial scientifically. Arguments which have been raised against that view are (i) that this entails a too-simplistic interpretation of the placebo effect (Freedman, 1997a, b); and (ii) that a placebo controlled trial only shows a treatment's efficacy against nothing, it does not shows its merits relative to other treatments (Freedman, 1997a, b; Aspinall and Goodman, 1995). The latter problem can be overcome by including active arms in a placebo controlled trial.

The duty-based approach, which will more often conclude that a trial should not be placebo controlled, would not do so for scientific reasons. Rather, the view is that it is simply wrong to deny treatments, if there are any, to patients who after all expect to be treated. For it is one thing to establish that, for scientific reasons, a trial needs a placebo arm. It is another for an individual researcher to be in equipoise about that placebo arm. For the duty-based approach to be satisfied, the researcher needs to be entirely happy that her patient will receive a placebo instead of an active treatment. This is not just a matter for science. The doctor has a series of responses to her patients which are neither mechanical nor capable of being anticipated. It may be, in some trials and for some patients, that a doctor will feel herself to be in equipoise about placebo. That is, she may feel it is as good for her patient to receive placebo as to receive an active treatment. There *is* a detectable placebo effect, and it may be that by avoiding the active arm the patient may also be avoiding noxious side effects. It is certainly true that patients do get better without active assistance from time to time. But there may be other cases where the doctor wants to take what Freedman calls a 'soft interpretation' of proven, available treatment. Then she may feel that a treatment which has become standard, even without having been proven against placebo, should be available to her patients in the trial who do not receive the experimental active treatment. In this case, active control equivalence studies would have to be designed. Collier (1995) argues that the gold standard against placebo should be established for every new drug, and the second generation of trials should no longer include placebo, but adopt the active control equivalence model. These are all possible answers to the fundamental challenge of therapeutic research on humans, but none is final.

My own conclusion is that duty-based morality, in the form of acting in a patient's best interests, should take priority, because the doctor's duty of care applies in every circumstance, whereas science *ought* to serve only ethical goals, and should compromise its rigour to that end. Otherwise, people become the servants of science inappropriately. The situation where the ultimate truth has been finally established about treatments for any condition is unlikely to be reached, if not ever, then certainly not for a very long time. Improvements will, indeed should, always be sought. If it is accepted as the norm that patients can be denied existing treatment for the sake of discovering the truth about the experimental treatment, that has to be recognized as a permanent feature of medical research. That, surely, is asking too much of patients? However, goal-based concerns, as they have shown themselves so far in this chapter, need to be taken seriously. The moral outlook of the doctor/researcher should always start with the duty to care for her patients, but it should stay open to the needs of all future patients too. She should not be prepared to compromise her own patients' needs but neither should she be ignorant of the need for rigorous research into new treatments. Finally, definitions of harm should guard against being over-cautious.

Non-therapeutic research

Duty to care versus scientific goals: potential risks in non-therapeutic research

The difficulties of balancing duty to care against science are challenging enough in therapeutic research, where patients are in trials with therapeutic intention and can expect their researching doctors to treat them as well as if they were patients in the ordinary way. Non-therapeutic research provides even more scope for having to make difficult decisions.

The question of whether or not to use placebo was a difficult one because of the duty-based need to ensure that patients in research projects were treated as well as possible. In non-therapeutic research, there is no intended therapeutic benefit, and there is always some risk of harm. The most difficult of all to justify are those studies where the subjects are not able to consent to take part. When a justification is found, it has to mean that the duty-based concern to do no harm, and the right-based concern only to act if the person affected agrees, have both been subsumed under the goal-based need to conduct the research. But the goal-based needs are considerable. Research into conditions which affect those who cannot consent needs to be done if treatments are to be developed. Some of that research will, of necessity, be non-therapeutic.

Research in a vulnerable group: trial into the causes of sudden infant death syndrome

A controversial study reported in 1998 highlights the moral difficulties (Parkins et al., 1998a). Sudden infant death syndrome is harrowing and one of its worst aspects is that its cause is unknown. Researchers at an academic department of paediatrics became interested in a possible cause when two sets of parents attended their outpatients' clinic reporting a child dying of sudden infant death syndrome shortly after having been on an intercontinental flight. The clinicians thought that a reduction in the partial pressure of inspired oxygen may increase the risk of apparent life-threatening events and sudden death in infancy. Airway hypoxia may be caused by respiratory tract infection or by a change to a higher altitude, such as air travel. In adults acute airway hypoxia has pronounced effects on the control of breathing during sleep. Very little is known about the effect of airway hypoxia on respiratory function in infants, but it is thought that the function would be more vulnerable to harm than adults.

The study exposed 34 infants to 15% oxygen in nitrogen (similar to the air in the cabin of a commercial aircraft) to discover the effects of airway hypoxia on arterial oxygenation and on the frequency of isolated and periodic apnoeic pauses. Twenty-one of the infants were from an obstetric unit run by a GP practice (mean age 3.1 months), and 13 were siblings of infants who had died from sudden infant death syndrome (mean age 1.8 months). Eligibility criteria included that the infants must have been born at term, and have had no history of respiratory distress or congenital anomalies.

The infants had an overnight recording of their oxygen saturation and respiratory variables in their own homes at room temperature and sea level air pressure. In terms of procedures the infants were put through, this meant a pulse oximeter (a cuff that is placed over a finger) and a volume expansion capsule placed on the abdominal wall (a tampon strapped to the baby's body). The recordings were analysed to ensure that the infant's heart rate and lung function were within normal limits before the infant was exposed to 15% oxygen. This took place on the second night in an oxygen tent at the paediatric unit. During this time the baby had the same measurements taken with the same instruments, and in addition, to monitor respired oxygen and carbon dioxide, a cannula was placed on the upper lip, which would have been fixed in place with a clip. A paediatrician remained with the infants during the period of exposure to 15% oxygen, and if the infant's oxygen saturation dropped to less than or equal to 80% for more than one minute, exposure ceased. Where this did happen, parents were advised not to take their baby on an aeroplane until it was at least 12 months old.

The result of the study showed a highly variable response to acute airway hypoxia. Some infants became so hypoxic they had to be withdrawn from exposure. It was not possible, however, from the previous measurements in room air at sea level air pressure, to predict which of the babies would suffer this effect. There may, then, be a relationship between hypoxic conditions and sudden infant death syndrome. The clinical implications of the study were recorded by the authors as follows:

We have shown that a small number of infants may become hypoxaemic during several hours of exposure to a fraction of inspired oxygen of 0.15 to 0.16. We could not, for ethical and humanitarian reasons, determine whether this would have progressed to clinically apparent cyanotic episodes [infant turning a greenish-blue] if exposure had continued. Unfortunately, there was no physiological or clinical variable in this study which would help identify infants who might develop clinically import-ant hypoxaemia during later exposure to airway hypoxia. We believe that additional research is urgently needed into the effects on infants of prolonged airline flights or holidays at high altitude. Our findings may contribute to an understanding of the possible relation between respiratory infection with resulting airway hypoxia and some sudden deaths in infancy.

The outcome of the research looks important. This study showed reliably that there was reason to be worried about the effect of air travel, and laid the foundations for future research. A goal-based analysis would find that it was necessary and morally justified. From a duty-based perspective, the research was designed so that the moment any distress was caused to the infant by virtue of its exposure, it was removed from the exposure. To that extent it honoured duty-based moral demands. But it is also true to say that it was not during the airline flight but afterwards that the infants whose untimely death had given rise to the researchers' hypothesis had in fact died, a point not picked up in the paper itself but noted by Savulescu who commented on it (Savulescu, 1998). So although the infants were carefully protected from harm during the study itself, they could not be protected from the risk of the consequences of what was done to them. For this important reason, the duty-based moralist will assert that the research should not have happened, or at any rate not using an experimental trial design.

It is often argued that the only way to research hypotheses about the bad consequences of risky behaviour is to use observational methods of research, for example, into the hypothesis that living near a busy traffic junction causes asthma in young children, or that smoking cigarettes causes lung cancer, because it would not be ethical to set up an experimental trial by, say, moving some children to live near a busy junction and seeing whether they contracted asthma or not. The fact that there is a concern with the risk of the exposure means that it can only be measured in an observational model. By contrast, the babies' deliberate exposure to 15% oxygen was an attempt to create the environment which the researchers believed may have been the cause of sudden infant death syndrome. The infants were placed in that environment in order to see what the effect was.

The goal-based justification for the research is not trivial. Sudden infant death syndrome remains a mystery and this research has provided a clue which may help to solve it. Such right-based concerns as could be met, were met by the parents giving their consent, a matter over which the researchers clearly took great care. But duty-based concerns about intentionally creating a risky environment were not treated as overriding. Rather, the goal-based need for sound science overrode the duty-based need to protect the babies from deliberate exposure to harm. If a proposal for non-therapeutic research is found to be acceptable it will be because the duty-based concerns have been subsumed by the goal-based scientific justification. If it is found not to be acceptable it will be because the duty-based concerns are so strong that they outweigh the goal-based need to conduct the research altogether. In this case, in my view, the duty-based concern should have been paramount.

However, the researchers themselves, the research ethics committee which approved the research, and the editor who published the results, clearly thought long and hard about the issues. The journal published the paper with the research findings, which itself included a discussion of the ethical issues (Parkins et al., 1998a), a commentary by Savulescu (1998), a commentary by the chairman of the research ethics committee which passed the proposal (Hughes, 1998), and the authors' reply to the two commentaries (Parkins et al., 1998b). Those concerned gave the matter considerable thought, and that must be respected.

My own final word is that the case supports the view that duty-based concerns should remain pre-eminent against goal-based ones. If the researchers had started with their duty of care to the infants as the moral basis for the research, they would have been more likely to think of using an observational design for the investigations.

Duty to care versus patient autonomy: non-therapeutic healthy volunteer research indicates the need to protect subjects from harm even if they consent

Healthy volunteer research is distinguishable by its use of healthy people, usually young men, as guinea pigs for research purposes. Most often it takes place within the pharmaceutical industry when new chemical entities are tried for the first time in humans (Phase I studies). These volunteers will be paid for their services. They will typically spend some time in Phase I research units, which, governed by comprehensive guidelines (ABPI, 1991), have proper facilities for care and resuscitation if necessary. Medical and nursing care are present and the experiments are conducted according to strict regulations (ICHGCP, 1997). Giving a new chemical entity to a human being carries numerous foreseeable and unforeseeable risks. Research will have been conducted in animals, but animals are not perfect models of humans, and much will still not be known about the toxicity of the novel entity, nor how the human body will digest and excrete it. The purpose of Phase I studies is to find these things out. Phase I studies do not seek to discover the therapeutic efficacy of the new drug. This waits until after the drug is known to be safe for humans to take.

Very toxic drugs such as chemotherapeutic agents for cancer treatment are not given to healthy volunteers because the toxicity levels are known to be high. Such drugs have to be tested in patients straightaway. That presents its own set of problems, since although the moral framework is clear, that the hoped-for benefit should outweigh the predicted risk, both risk and benefit are hypothetical, and so the actual decision is very difficult indeed. It is made more difficult by the fact that patients will often have tried every other treatment option and may accept, in their desperation, anything which holds out only very tiny chances of helping, even when the risks are very high indeed (McBride, 1994).

Most new chemical entities, however, start by being studied in healthy volunteers and these trials are transparently non-therapeutic. Because the volunteers are healthy adults it is possible to have a very clear understanding with them that there is no therapeutic intention in the trial and that there will be some risk. Information sheets can be long and detailed, because there need be no concern that these participants will be feeling too ill to go through them carefully and think about what they are being told. Volunteers are also expected to be honest about their own medical and social history, so that the researchers can reject any for whom participation in their trial would be unwise or even medically dangerous. Participants, as was said, are paid.

Healthy volunteer study of eproxindine hydrochloride, 1985

In 1985 shock waves went through the clinical research community and research ethics committees when the death of a healthy volunteer was reported (Darragh et al., 1985). The medical examination he had been given had not picked up, and he had not spoken of, a depot injection of flupen-thixol on the day before his death. The study was of eproxindine hydrochloride, a new anti-arrhythmic agent. The study was designed to investigate tolerance of humans to single, rising, intravenous doses of the drug given by infusion over five minutes. One hundred and ninety-two doses had already been given over a period of seven months to healthy young men using the same routes, and no adverse reactions had been seen. This young man, however, had a sudden cardiorespiratory arrest and died. Afterwards it became known 'from non-medical sources' that he had attended a psychiatric outpatient clinic where he had received an injection, which was, as subsequent blood tests showed, of flupenthixol. Although the precise mechanism for the interaction between the study drug and flupenthixol is not known, both are basic drugs and are highly protein bound.

The young man, together with all the other participants, had been told that all medicines, illicit social drugs, and alcohol were prohibited throughout the study. At no time did the volunteer who died admit to receiving any medication, nor did he disclose information relating to his recent medical history. He had first attended the clinic as a healthy volunteer six years previously, and had participated in about two studies per year since then. He had been independently examined by eight different physicians, none of whom had detected the condition and treatment which would have excluded him from being a participant in the trials at the clinic. As the authors of the report point out, the case highlights the difficulties of screening out volunteers. Without full disclosure of the medical history, most comprehensive medical examinations and tests will be inadequate.

'Kidology'

A story told in the *British Medical Journal* in 1998 rather nicely illustrates the need to guard against over-eager and mendacious healthy volunteers, who assume that, being in the hands of doctors and research ethics committees, they will not come to any harm.

The train journey, the pile of papers, and the *BMJ*. The man opposite catches my eye.
    'I see you're a doctor.'
    Self – aiming at closure: 'Yes, I've a lot of work to get through.'
    'I'm on my way back from London. I was in Harley Street being interviewed as a volunteer for a drug trial of antidepressants. I had to use some "kidology".'
    'Yes?'
    'I'm not depressed but they pay better in London than they do in Scotland or Manchester but I don't think I succeeded. The doctor advised me to use cognitive therapy. They said they would pay my expenses by cheque but eventually agreed to give me cash.'
    'Oh?'
    'Yes, the trials are advertised, the best pay about £100 a day to volunteers. For a 20 day trial that's £2000. The worst trial was when I had to be woken up every hour to do mental tests, but usually it's like being on a health farm.'
    'What about making sure you don't come to harm?'
    'Oh, they have a committee of vicars and lawyers to decide it's all right, and it's nice to see your regular friends.'
    My train drew into the station; I was no longer irritated at the interruption. (Boyd, 1998)

Audit of volunteer screening procedures

An audit of the screening procedures for healthy volunteers reported in 1992 showed the importance of obtaining reports on the volunteers from their GPs (Watson and Wyld, 1992). Information so received revealed important facts not disclosed during the medical history or examination of the healthy volunteers themselves. The audit was of the rejection rate and stage at which rejection took place in 831 subjects all volunteering for the same study. The screening procedure at this unit was in three stages: first, the volunteers filled out a questionnaire with personal, social and medical details; at this stage 117 of the 831 were rejected. Second, a medical history was taken, and a physical examination performed with clinical chemistry and haematology investigations and serology for Hepatitis B and HIV. A urine sample was tested for protein, glucose, blood and bilirubin, and also for drugs of abuse. At this stage 45 volunteers were rejected. Stage three consisted of obtaining information from the GP of each of the volunteers. The questionnaire the GP was asked to complete asked about disorders of the central nervous system, cardiovascular disorders, disorders of the respiratory system, disorders and diseases of the alimentary system and the genito-urinary system, psychiatric disorders, alcohol and/or drug abuse, and any other disorders such as diabetes mellitus. The GP was asked about any prescribed drugs and evidence of adverse drug reactions, and about the involvement of his patient in any previous research studies within the last six months. The GP was asked if there was any reason he felt the volunteer should not participate in the research. Finally, he was asked how long his records went back on the volunteer in question. At this stage 44 more volunteers were rejected.

On the basis of information from GPs, four volunteers were rejected for depressive illness, 18 for alcohol dependency, four for drug dependency, and six for neurological disorders (including one case of epilepsy and four of recent head injuries, two of whom had been prescribed prophylactic anticonvulsant drugs). The understated conclusion of the authors is: 'Application to the GP for medical information on potential volunteers is an important step in the screening of volunteer subjects for clinical research'.

Does payment to research subjects make a moral difference?

In healthy volunteer studies, the research participants are in a much better position than patients for the purposes of obtaining consent. They are healthy and competent, and there is no need to rush the consent procedure. We could think that the duty-based approach becomes redundant in these trials, for if the science is good (goal-based) and the subjects are fully consenting, that is to say, are perfectly well aware of any risk (right-based), there are no other moral concerns. However, the mendacity about social or medical habits indicated in the audit of volunteer screening procedures was almost certainly due to the lure of money, which affected the exercising of their judgement, thus raising a question mark over the validity of the right-based criterion being met. It can be assumed that the reason individuals choose to take part in healthy volunteer studies is that they would like the remuneration offered. But in many other circumstances individuals are paid for doing risky jobs, such as city couriers, stuntmen and women, and security guards. Is there a difference between those situations and that of the healthy volunteer who knowingly takes a risk for money?

The additional factors in the medical research context that may make a difference are the presence of healthcare professionals and the reference to a research ethics committee. The potential healthy volunteer may or may not be aware of the latter (the depressive *manqué* was) but he will certainly know about the former because they are conducting the trial. He may assume that the researcher will not do anything that will harm him, even if he is told that she will. To this extent the research must honour the duty-based moral requirement not to be too risky. It would be wrong to propose risky research and let the prospect of payment lure the healthy volunteer to accept those risks when, as I say, he will have a belief that a doctor would not deliberately expose him to harm. But only the volunteer himself can be held responsible for lying about social and medical habits that will expose him to risks if he continues with them and also enters the trial. The lure of money may encourage mendacity but for that no-one can or should be held accountable but the volunteer himself.

Women of child-bearing potential as healthy volunteers

Until recently, women of child-bearing potential, that is, healthy young women, were routinely excluded from Phase I studies because of the risk to the fetus if they were by some chance pregnant. Hence, healthy volunteer studies were almost always on young men. This reflected a duty-based concern. It meant that data from Phase I studies were always based upon studying male participants. The difference, of course, is that whereas a man is taking a risk just with his own body, the woman will be taking a risk both with her own body and with the fetus. However, it seems inconsistent not to rely on a woman knowing that she is pregnant and disclosing that information for the fetus' safety, when researchers have to rely on a man's honesty about his drinking and other social habits.

Summary and concluding remarks

In this chapter some examples have been considered where the duty-based considerations of acting in the patients' best interests weigh sufficiently in the balance as to force either goal-based or right-based assumptions to be reconsidered. The primary goal-based assumption brought into question is that it is of overriding importance that the science of a research project is as pure as possible. The primary right-based assumption is that if people have been fully informed of what they are to consent to, are competent, and have given their voluntary agreement, then they have a right to go forward to be a research participant.

In considering the issue of scientific rigour the use of placebo controls in therapeutic research was discussed. The arguments on both sides were investigated, seeing how a goal-based thinker, such as Ciociola, tries to show that the scientifically rigorous trial is also in accordance with a duty-based ethic, because patients would come to no real harm and could be excluded if there was any possibility that they would. We saw how a duty-based thinker, such as Freedman, tries to show that trials which honour the duty of care to patients can also be scientifically rigorous. Examples of trials in which the use of placebo was contentious were looked at: folic acid in pregnancy; trials of peptic ulcer disease; and ondansetron trials. It was noted in conclusion that whilst goal-based and duty-based approaches might reach out to each other, they do not, in fact, meet in the middle. It was suggested that for this reason it was important to put the duty-based duty of care in primary place, but at the same time remain open to the need to conduct scientifically rigorous trials, and then let each case stand on its own merits.

A more worrying example of a trial in which the goal-based considerations overrode duty-based ones was then described and analysed. This was the trial of babies, exposed to the same atmospheric conditions of an inter-continental aeroplane. Although the immediate risk was not great, and indeed mimicked atmospheric conditions into which babies are introduced every time their parents fly with them, the conditions were thought to contribute to sudden infant death syndrome, so the longer-term risk was considerable, and unknown. The researchers created an ideal experimental situation, which produced a scientifically satisfactory result, when they should have used the less rigorous observational model of research which is employed when investigating other sorts of risky behaviour, such as smoking. Goal-based considerations had overridden duty-based ones in an inappropriate way. If the researchers had started from the duty-based foundation of not harming their research participants, rather than starting with the need for scientific rigour and considering the safety of the babies only secondarily (with however much care), they would have been more likely to propose a different trial design, such as an observational one. I am not suggesting that the researchers did not take the risks to the babies sufficiently seriously, because clearly they thought long and hard about the issue. What I am suggesting is that the notion of not harming was not the prior consideration. It came after the research was designed. From a duty-based starting point, other research design possibilities might have opened up, as has been discussed. Without such a basis, they were not even mentioned.

Finally, an example of duty-based morality clashing with right-based morality was considered. The evidence from the audit of screening potential healthy volunteers through their doctors was that to rely on a person's self-selection in this situation will mean that some individuals will go forward as volunteers who should not. On the presumption that the individuals volunteer because of the money involved, such remuneration should never be for undergoing risk and researchers should live up to the expectation that they would not deliberately cause harm. However, mendacity about social habits cannot be the responsibility of anyone but the liar, even if he is being paid.

The discussion in this chapter has focused on the duty-based issue of the doctor/researcher's duty of care to her research subjects, which demands that she acts in their best interests. This need comes into conflict with both goal-based issues of scientific validity, and right-based issues of patient autonomy. In seeking to come to a reasonable conclusion when faced with this conflict it was proposed that the duty-based perspective remains pre-eminent, in the sense that that is where each doctor should start. However, the goal-based moral demands are sufficiently strong to warrant serious attention from every doctor. Therefore, while staying with her duty to care for each of her patients, each doctor must remain open to the need to be continually developing new treatments and improving old ones. The doctor is concerned for the patient she is currently treating, *and* for all those in the future who will need care. The danger of the duty-based approach being arrogant, because of the doctor's necessary assumption of knowing what is in her patients' best interests, is tempered by the right-based demand that she seek to know and respect the views of her potential research participants. Whilst she might need to question a healthy volunteer's eagerness to be her research participant, she should certainly not question his refusal. It is to issues of consent as they have arisen in particular cases that we now turn.

8

Case studies of right-based issues

Introduction

This chapter will look at the practical application of right-based morality in research on humans, which is expressed as the need to obtain consent and to respect confidentiality. These are the two primary moral demands of right-based morality, as I have defined it. By consent is meant the adequately informed, voluntary agreement of a competent person to participate in research. By confidentiality is meant the non-disclosure of private information which has been given in a medical context, where no consent to disclosure has been given or can be assumed.

When consent and confidentiality were discussed at a theoretical level it was argued that they were essential moral requirements. In the context of particular cases, goal-based demands for rigorous science and duty-based demands to act in a patient's best interests also weigh in the balance. I propose to consider the right-based requirement for consent in the face of goal-, duty- and, paradoxically, right-based obstacles to its being successfully obtained. Empirical studies of the consent procedure for these purposes will be concentrated on. The extent to which the use of consent forms can be regarded as helping or hindering the consent process will also be considered. Under confidentiality one argument against respecting it, which arises from the goal-based need to conduct records-based research, will be considered.

Consent

Consent to participation in research is demanded by the right-based principle, that no person should be treated merely as a means to an end, but always also as an end in herself. The idea that anyone is merely expendable is abhorrent; it has given rise to such atrocities as those committed by the Nazis in concentration camps, or by the injustice of apartheid in South Africa. That anyone should be expendable for the *good* of others or in the service of a greater good (as in being a research participant) does not make it any more right. The Nazis and the government of South Africa thought they were acting for a greater good. It does not follow, however, that no-one *should* be used in the service of others. The significant additional factor that makes the use morally acceptable is that each person *agrees* that she is so used. It is one thing to be forced to serve others and quite another willingly to do so. The latter is to be highly recommended. In medical research this means that consent should always be sought.

Nevertheless, there are numerous ways in which the consent process can be undermined in the context of research. Some of these attacks are effective. To illustrate this, right-based, duty-based and goal-based constraints on the consent process will be looked at, starting with right-based concerns because they could be said to be among the most difficult to answer. Duty-based and goal-based concerns, whilst compelling, could be overruled by using right-based morality as a trump card. Thus, the response would be given that no matter, for example, that the giving of information to a person in order to seek her consent will cause her distress (a duty-based concern), it is nevertheless more important that she is informed and makes up her own mind. Alternatively, the response could be, if the obtaining of consent means that important research will be severely curtailed because of low recruitment (a goal-based concern), that again, it is still more important that people are not used merely as a means to an end. Right-based morality is the basis of the demand that consent be sought, so if it presents difficulties in obtaining consent, these cannot be answered so easily.

Right-based difficulties with consent: the empirical evidence

There are numerous opinions about what the consent procedure needs to consist of if it is to succeed. The relentless disagreement between different research ethics committees and between research ethics committees and researchers on this point alone is sufficient witness to this fact. Rather than rehearse the disagreements, some empirical studies which highlight some of the difficulties will be looked at. There are clearly more studies of this area than there is room to discuss here, but a good spread of studies will be referred to, hopefully giving a fair picture.

Patients felt they were well-informed

First, there is a positive result from a study conducted some time ago (Goodman et al., 1984). This research surveyed patients from two trials which were studying the ventilatory effects of postoperative analgesia. There were 18 patients in each of the trials. Fourteen out of the 18 patients in the first study returned questionnaires; 18 out of 18 returned questionnaires in the second study. In the first study the questionnaire was sent to all 18 patients who had completed the postoperative phase of the study. In the second study the questionnaire was given to patients after the operation but before they were discharged from hospital.

The results were promising for the success of the consent procedure: of the

32 respondents, 30 thought the explanation prior to their giving consent was satisfactory. Eleven had felt obliged to participate in the trial, but not from any feeling of coercion, but rather from a sense of duty to others. Of the eight who found discomfort from the operation, only one felt that it was worse than the prior explanation had given him to believe.

King's review of the literature

Other studies, however, have not been so positive in their findings. Jennifer King (1986) undertook a review of the empirical research on the consent procedure; her findings are mixed, to say the least. One observation from the review was that patients' needs and wishes for information are generally greater than many doctors realize or cater for, although, as King points out, the degree of information wanted will inevitably vary with the individual patient and the condition she suffers from. She quotes one researcher's conclusion: 'To tell or not to tell is not the issue, but rather what information is appropriate for a particular patient' (Hoy, 1985).

Three studies in the review showed a failure of patients properly to understand what they had been told (Garnham, 1975; Leeb et al., 1976; Cassileth et al., 1980). However, the method in these studies relied on patients' recall of what they had been told, in some cases after a few months had elapsed. This is not really a measure of the patients' understanding at the time: there are plenty of situations in which we take in information, understand it and act upon it, and then forget about it soon afterwards. Four other studies showed more success in helping patients' understanding when certain strategies and communication techniques were adopted to improve information giving (Ley, 1979; Woodward, 1979; Holtzman et al., 1983; Simes et al., 1986).

Other studies reviewed by King show duty- and goal-based problems, which will be turned to under those headings. Obviously, a number of studies have been conducted since 1986, and some of these will be looked at now.

Volunteers tend to be less well-educated

In 1990, a sad but unsurprising finding was reported in Australia: that parents who volunteer their children for research are less well-educated, and hold fewer administrative or professional jobs than those who do not. Their motivation is to help others, but it also comes from a desire to gain more information and to help their own children (Harth and Thong, 1990).

Patients do not understand information sheets

Another study in 1990 was even more depressing, giving reasons to believe that patients do not understand what they are told, no matter how hard clinicians try to make written information comprehensible (Sutherland et al., 1990). An information sheet and consent form for a hypothetical trial was given to patients. The inclusion criteria were: all patients had been admitted to one hospital requiring postsurgical treatment for cancer; they all knew they were being treated for cancer; they all understood written and spoken English; they all gave consent to participate. The study excluded patients who had previously consented or refused to enter a clinical trial, or who had undergone chemotherapy. Patients were asked to underline the information on the sheet which was pertinent to their decision to take part in the hypothetical study. Seventy-four per cent did not indicate that both risks and benefits were pertinent. Twenty out of 50 refused to take part in the study; for 70% of those, only information about risks was pertinent to their decision. Thirty out of 50 agreed; for 33% of those, the only information pertinent to them was about risks, while 10% noted neither benefits nor risks. This part of the results indicates only that different patients are moved by or want to know about different information, a finding already established. However, the researchers also gave patients a multiple choice test of the meaning of four of the statements in the information sheet. Between 26% and 54% of the answers, depending on the statement, were wrong. One of the statements was 'a particular type of cancer responds to radiation treatment in 10% of cases'. Forty-six per cent of respondents thought, correctly, that that meant: 'on average, for 10 out of every 100 patients, the tumour will decrease in size after radiation treatment'. But 22% thought it meant: 'the radiation treatment is about 10% effective in an individual patient'. Another 22% thought it meant: '10% of patients are cured'. Ten per cent thought it meant: 'there is a 10% chance of survival'. Another of the statements read: 'a process called randomization is used to select your treatment in this clinical trial'. Sixty-eight per cent, correctly, thought that meant: 'each individual patient has exactly the same chance of receiving the drug, or not receiving the drug, as any other participating patient'. But 14% thought it meant: 'the process will select the best treatment for me', and 18% thought it meant: 'the doctor decides which treatment is the right one for me'. The lack of understanding of randomization is supported by findings in later studies which I shall come to shortly.

Benefits remembered more than risks

A report in the *British Medical Journal* of a study in Chicago indicated that cancer patients enrolled in a Phase I trial do not take in much of the information given to them prior to agreeing to take part. Only one third correctly thought the study was of dose escalation; the other two thirds did not know or thought it was therapeutic. The *British Medical Journal*, citing the researcher who conducted the survey, observed:

Clearly, despite attempts at explanations, patients' motivation to get some therapeutic benefit is so overwhelming that it obliterates the memories of much of what they have been told about the study. (McBride, 1994)

This worrying finding is partly explained by the research of Slevin and others (1990) which found that people who actually had cancer 'are much more likely to opt for radical treatment with minimal chance of benefit than people who do not have cancer, including medical and nursing professionals'. In 1994, Chee Saw and others found that patients were more likely to remember the benefits they had been told about than the risks (Chee Saw et al., 1994). The information was about the transurethral resection of the prostate which patients were about to undergo: the risk of retrograde ejaculation was stressed when the information was given, and yet 18% of patients did not remember that this was one of the risks, when they were asked. This selective remembering of only the better news was found in another study (McDaniel Hutson and Blaha, 1991).

Randomization not really understood: the ECMO study

Qualitative methods were used (Snowdon et al., 1997) to explore in detail parental reactions to random allocation of treatment in an important national neonatal trial: the UK collaborative trial of extra-corporeal membrane oxygenation (ECMO). The trial involved mature newborn babies with acute, but potentially reversible, respiratory failure, comparing conventional management, that is, maximal ventilatory support, with a novel treatment, ECMO, which involved oxygenation of the blood via an external circuit. The ECMO treatment meant the baby would be attached to the ECMO circuit by an operation to insert cannulae into blood vessels in the neck. The treatment also often involved a journey by air ambulance since there were only five centres in the UK with the equipment. ECMO had been widely adopted elsewhere in the world, though not subject to properly controlled trials. In Britain, by dint of careful collaboration, the trial of ECMO involved paediatric units right across the country, and ECMO was only available in the trial.

The research by Snowdon and others explored parents' understanding of randomization. Three observations should be made about the study before looking at those findings which have implications for right-based problems with consent. First, the parents concerned were in an extremely stressful situation with a newborn baby who was critically ill and needed treatment quickly. Second, although parents were given letters and information leaflets about the trial which had been prepared by the trial steering committee, some centres were required by local research ethics committees to amend or replace the trial documentation, and in some instances to use locally idiosyncratic consent forms. Additional information would have been given to parents at the discretion of the participating centres' staff, since they were asked to expand on the written information. Hence, the basic information given to parents was not uniform. Third, there was widespread belief amongst parents that ECMO was the superior treatment.

For 12 of the 21 pairs of parents interviewed, at least one of the parents understood the nature of randomization. Of those who did not, some saw the treatment decision as therapeutic:

Andrea based her understanding on information she was given about her son's eligibility for the trial. When the possibility of the trial was raised with Andrea and Robert, Daniel did not quite fulfil the entry criteria, but would do so if he deteriorated further. She found this difficult to explain and eventually concluded that, although Daniel was dying, he still needed to decline to a stage where conventional therapy would be of no assistance.

When asked about their perceptions of how randomization was actually carried out, most parents were aware that a computer was involved; some thought it was to make a more sophisticated treatment decision, others to generate a simple binary decision. One parent, interestingly, described the process of minimization (a refined version of randomization in which the computer will ensure the groups are comparable according to pre-set data, which was used in this trial) but without describing the random element. The woman said:

It would be randomly selection from like a computer . . . We assumed that what would happen is . . . that the information . . . would have been fed through the computer and that I assume that if they had em already had information on a baby girl, round eight pound to nine pound weight, and they had already had on ECMO trial, then they would do the other . . . I thought that perhaps the reason we didn't go onto the ECMO trial was because they already had somebody, or previously had somebody, same weight, same sex, similar problem.

The authors report that by contrast to this account, other parents said they had received very simple information, such as that the child's name only went into the computer:

How they always put it was the button would be pressed and if his name came up he would be gone [i.e. transferred for ECMO].

The authors observe that the comment reflected a belief that several babies were competing for ECMO places; an understanding of the random decision but a distortion of the reasons for making the decision randomly. Another couple were given conflicting information: that only the child's name would be fed into the computer; and that the child's details would be fed in.

When asked about the reasons for randomization, only four parents suggested methodological reasons, for example the need in research for controls. This was typical of how parents viewed the conventional treatment:

You canna really do a trial if you put them all on to it . . . You've got to leave some to compare it against.

Most parents described ethical reasons for randomization in a more-or-less muddled way. A number saw it as a way of not asking the doctors to play God in allocating a limited resource. Robert, whose son had gone into the ECMO arm, said:

I just felt there could have been ten other babies with exactly the same problems as him and now there is nine sets of parents who are now being told that their baby's not being accepted onto the trial. And I did feel a bout of guilt for that but I could have gone out and ... danced on water ... when I got told that he'd been accepted.

Most parents were uncomfortable with randomization and only one said it was important to 'test properly' the new treatment; only one other suggested it was necessary to randomize in order to assess ECMO for associated hazards. A number regarded the process as unfair or tough and heartless:

I suppose trials have to be a bit heartless, but you'd think that when the baby looks like they're dying, you'd think they'd just say ... 'Oh hell' you know 'let's try the ECMO, see if it saves this baby', but with that sort of a trial they can't do that can they? They have to say, 'Well look, this baby looks like it's dying but I'm sorry it's getting conventional treatment and that's that'.

Many accounts of parents convey a sense that randomization was a trivial way to make a choice. A doctor should be expected to be more careful and considered in how he decided.

Robert felt that ECMO was a proven treatment and so should not be restricted. When he was asked what he was told about how the treatment would be chosen:

Yes, by randomisation and that – that annoyed me. It didn't annoy me at the time because we got it [ECMO] but since then the very thing that's stuck in my mind all the time is who gives them the right to play God with babies' lives? And why the hell have we got it on trial when it's been in the States and it's got an 89% success rate or whatever ... ? Why is the National Health playing around with this? You know they wouldn't play around if America suddenly came up with a cure for cancer ... Why are they playing around with babies' lives? Er, you know who gives them the right to sit here with say 10 babies and think well this – this one here you know will – will suit the trial, you know. Why not all 10 of them? Why isn't it available everywhere so everybody has a fair chance?

This study gives an insight into the meaning of randomization to lay people. Randomization is not generally very well understood, and people do not appreciate that the doctors may genuinely not know which is the better treatment, or indeed that ECMO was not proven to be effective. The widespread belief, clearly shown in these responses, that ECMO was the superior treatment, would have made a big impact on the ability or willingness of the parents to comprehend randomization. Whether or not there was strong equipoise in the doctors' minds, there was clearly no such balance of uncertainty in the minds of the parents. This is a good demonstration of the problems with communication that the consent procedure has to overcome if it is to be more than a semblance of the real thing.

There are further, related questions to ponder. Does it matter that the parents may well have agreed to enrol their babies into the ECMO trial not because of the uncertainty of which of the two treatments was better, but because it was the only way their baby had any chance at all of receiving ECMO, since it was not offered outside the trial? If ECMO had been available without having to enrol in the trial, would the vast majority of parents have refused to enter their babies for the trial and opted for ECMO instead? If so, the ECMO trial would never have been able to happen and the superiority of ECMO would not have been established with scientific rigour. This is a goal-based imperative. By only being offered ECMO in the trial, however, parents were not really making a voluntary choice about enrolling their babies, they were being coerced on the basis of their beliefs about ECMO. Does the fact that they may have been wrong about ECMO's superiority make the coercion morally acceptable? That is to say, the parents may have felt an obligation to enter their babies into the trial because that was the only way they could be sure they were doing the best they could for their child, and therefore their consent was not really valid, because it felt to them that they *had* no choice. But because the basis for their sense of obligation was objectively wrong (that ECMO was indubitably the superior treatment), the parents actually made the right decision, albeit for the wrong reason, because no one was worse off on the basis of it (the babies' best interests were served, which is the duty-based imperative) and the future surgical care of babies in their condition was helped (the goal-based imperative). But what then of the right-based imperative that we should be of service to others only by our free will?

It seems to me that this conundrum is a fact of life in many circumstances other than medical research on humans. My reasons for agreeing to certain ways of being treated are always going to be mixed and based upon a less than perfect understanding of the facts. This is not a trivial observation, because in ethics, motive matters a great deal. We do not think morality is well served if we try to justify lack of understanding by asserting that, actually, our decision is objectively right. But motive can be separated from understanding. That is to say, the desire of the parents to do the best for their babies, regardless of how they came to understand how to do that, can be applauded. Indeed, had ECMO been available outside the trial, given the state of their beliefs about it, it would have been questionable if they *had* put their babies into the trial. By extension, if the research project was one where consent was not given vicariously but on a person's own behalf, the motive to help others could be applauded if it played a part in the decision of the individual to enter the trial.

Duty-based difficulties with consent

The theoretical difficulty that duty-based morality poses for consent is that it causes harm. In the above example of the ECMO study, the duty-based moralist might argue that none of these difficulties would have arisen if the parents had simply not been told that their babies were in a trial, or if they had been pre-randomized, with only those who had been randomized to ECMO being asked if they would like their child to be in the study. This circumvents the difficulty; it does not solve it, and is anathema to the right-based moralist whose response to the misconceptions of the parents is to try and improve communication with them, certainly not to conclude that consent should therefore not be sought. But there are compelling reasons for the duty-based approach to be taken seriously, even if, in the end, it is rejected.

Empirical evidence of whether information increases anxiety
One area that has been the subject of study is whether giving information increases anxiety, and what is the psychological/physiological effect of giving information to patients for the purposes of seeking their consent. King's 1986 review looked at some studies of this. Her conclusion was that it depends upon the patient, the condition, and the way in which information is given. There is certainly some evidence that information about side effects of treatment can lead to those side effects being experienced (e.g. Cairns et al., 1985). There is also evidence, however, that giving information can improve patients' recovery (Wallace, 1984, 1986). Kerrigan and others (1993) observed that 'detailed information did not increase patient anxiety' in men undergoing elective inguinal hernia repair. However, in Chee Saw et al.'s study (1994) referred to above, 54% of respondents did not want detailed explanations, trusting in the doctor to give them the right treatment.

Patients' consent should not automatically be sought in therapeutic research
An article by Tobias and Souhami (1993), which was, in duty-based fashion, entitled 'Informed consent can be needlessly cruel', cites arguments and evidence that often slip into goal-based reasoning (so the article might have been called: 'Informed consent prevents good clinical research'), which will be examined below. They do, however, make some duty-based points about the effect of the consent process on the patient. Their most significant point is that the double standard that currently exists between therapeutic research and treatment should go, and that the decision whether or not to inform a patient about what is happening to her should be based, in both situations, on her psychological and physiological state. The underlying premise is that

the clinical trial is as therapeutic for the patient as treatment in the ordinary way, since the trial is comparing new and standard treatments, and patients have a 50% chance of receiving the better treatment. The doctor does not know which it is, and therefore it is in accordance with his duty of care to his patient to put her in the trial. If in his view the patient would be unduly distressed by information, then, as he would if he were offering treatment in the ordinary way, he should withhold information, but still enrol her in the trial, because that is doing what he believes is best for her. Tobias and Souhami think that patients, when they are told what is wrong with them, particularly when it is a condition as frightening as cancer, want reassurance and a clear prognosis, not to be told that their doctor does not know what is best. They point out that in the consultation and discussion of the trial the doctor may describe the advantages of the experimental treatment, only to have to back peddle if the patient is then randomized to the conventional therapy arm. Although the right-based moralist would argue that it was the doctor's fault for enthusing about the novel treatment when he was supposed to be in equipoise, we can see from the ECMO trial findings and the Chee Saw study that it is not so easy to convey a balanced picture. Tobias and Souhami pick up the point that is demonstrated in the ECMO findings, that patients are disturbed by the knowledge that a computer, not a doctor, will be 'making the decision' about their treatment.

Problems with this argument

Right-based moralists would argue that people need to be informed, ought to be informed, and if that is at the price of their peace of mind then that is a price that must be paid. There *is* a difference between the ordinary therapeutic situation and that of the clinical trial, from the point of view of the patient, because in the ordinary situation (as the patient believes) the doctor knows what to do for her. In the context of research the doctor does not know, and the patient is helping him to find out for the sake of future patients. Were she to find out later that this is what had happened without her knowledge or consent, she would not be best pleased. Nor would she be inclined to trust her doctor in the future. From the patient's perspective, she has been deceived, and she has also been made to be of service to others without her consent. Tobias, Souhami, Chalmers (personal communication, 2000), Baum (1986, 1993) and others will argue that in the ordinary clinical situation the patient is also deceived because the doctor does not recognize that there are other treatment options. So there is deceit in both circumstances, but at least in the context of a trial some good is being achieved for future patients. The right-based perspective looks from the patient's eyes, however, and from here, the trial and the treatment situations are different because in the former the doctor would knowingly deceive the patient if he did not seek her consent, whereas in the latter the doctor is also in the dark and no deliberate deceit has been practised. The issue is, again, one of motive rather than objective fact, or what works out for the best in the end.

Lord Scarman's prudent patient test
Lord Scarman, who was one of the judges involved in the Sidaway v Bethlem Royal Hospital Governors (Sidaway, 1985), commented later:

> Even before *Sidaway* I was troubled – and I remain now very puzzled – as to the ethical and legal implications of the so-called randomised clinical trial, where, *ex hypothesi*, the doctor does not know, and is 'using', to put it baldly, his patient for the purposes of very worthwhile experimentation... As the law stands at the moment, I would have thought that any doctor who allows his patient to go into a randomised clinical trial without telling him runs a very real risk if things go wrong and the patient suffers injury or damage... One can see the value of this form of experimentation ... but I am bound to say that I think there is a danger for the doctor in going ahead with subjecting, if that is the correct word, his patient to a randomised clinical trial without warning him. (Scarman, 1986)

Goal-based difficulties with consent

The goal-based argument against consent is that seeking consent from patients reduces recruitment rates into trials to the extent that the trials themselves are in jeopardy. It is this conclusion at which Tobias and Souhami arrive when they state:

> The issue of informed consent has thus become a major barrier to the successful conduct of randomised clinical trials in cancer. The many practical difficulties have led to low levels of recruitment, especially where there is a substantial difference between the treatment policies being compared (Tobias and Souhami, 1993)

Empirical evidence that consent reduces recruitment
There is some empirical evidence to support their concerns. The development from duty-based to goal-based arguments in their article is rational given that one of the reasons that recruitment levels are low, apart from patients not wanting to join trials once they have been informed, is the reluctance of their doctors to talk to them about randomization (Taylor et al., 1984). This is, presumably, out of concern for their patients' well being, although, as one correspondent pointed out, it may be that the doctor is simply transferring his anxiety about challenging the efficacy of a new product to his patient (Walsworth-Bell, 1993).

The ISIS Trial in the United Kingdom and the United States
Tobias and Souhami cite the experience of the international study of infarct survival (ISIS) investigators. The second ISIS trial, ISIS II, studied streptokinase and aspirin in acute myocardial infarction. The patients who were

eligible for this trial were, therefore, extremely ill and in no fit state to give consent to participate. They were, in other words, incompetent at the time when consent would need to be sought. Nevertheless, what Collins described as 'humanly inappropriate' written informed consent conditions were demanded of the investigators in the United States. These led to a very poor recruitment rate compared with the UK, where 'consent' was permitted to be sought in whatever way was best for the patient (Collins et al., 1992). This was usually retrospective or sometimes, I regret to say, not taken at all. In the lengthy correspondence which followed the publication of Tobias' and Souhami's article many opinions were expressed on the matter, but some were able to give actual examples of the goal-based problems consent had caused. These were not only related to poor recruitment rate but also to the validity of the research results:

We recently had to relax the time between the diagnosis of breast cancer and recruitment to a study of adjuvant treatment. Because of observations that bisphosphonates decreased morbidity due to bone metastases in patients with breast cancer we wished to determine whether these agents might delay the appearance of skeletal disease when given to women at the time that breast cancer was diagnosed. We intended to test the intervention at the earliest possible time in the natural course of the disease, whereas the trauma to patients resulting from the diagnosis, radiotherapy, chemotherapy, and informed consent have permitted us to randomise our patients only up to six months after diagnosis (Kanis and Bergmann, 1993).

The breast conservation trial and the President's Commission
In King's 1986 review the United Kingdom breast conservation trial is cited as an example of a trial which had to be stopped due to poor recruitment following information given to patients (*British Medical Journal*, 1983). However, the President's Commission study which aimed to identify reasons for refusal of treatment found that the outstanding reason for refusal was bad communication (President's Commission, 1983).

Patients will not happily agree to being randomized
More pertinently for our discussion, the Simes et al. (1986) study already referred to found that the better informed the patients were, the less likely they were to agree to randomization. This seems to be because the tendency to want to establish a preference for one or other treatment is stronger than the acceptance of genuine uncertainty.

Research which cannot take place if consent is sought
Finally, there are those research projects which could not happen at all if consent were to be sought, not because difficulties in obtaining consent scupper recruitment, but because the outcome of the research depends upon

the subjects not knowing they are in a trial. One such example (McArdle et al., 1996), was a study of different levels of psychological support for women following breast cancer surgery. Varying levels of support from diverse sources (routine care; routine care and breast care nurse; routine care and support organization; routine care, nurse and support organization) were compared with each other to see which was the most beneficial. The research showed that morbidity was consistently lower in the group which received care from the breast care nurse only.

If the women concerned had known that they were participating in a research project, their responses to the support would have been affected and would have rendered the study scientifically invalid. The goal-based requirements demanded that the right-based requirements were waived. My own comment on the research at the time was this:

Does this [not obtaining consent in order to conduct the research] make the trial unethical? The answer to this question depends on the balance of apparently competing moral claims. If you regard the research question as paramount you might argue that the need to do the research outweighed the moral requirement to consult the subjects of the research. If you regard the subjects' welfare as paramount then you would be happy in this case since the subjects would suffer no harm. But if your overriding concern is that the wishes of people being used as a means to someone else's ends should first be consulted then you would not consider this research to be ethical. By extension, of course, any research which needed to deceive the research subjects in order to obtain a result would not be regarded as ethical. (Foster, 1996)

Interjection: should research be published if it was conducted unethically?

Both the study of infants in high-altitude tents (see Chapter Seven), and the study of post-operative support for breast cancer patients, involved waiving important moral principles, the former of a duty-based nature, the latter of a goal-based nature. A question often pondered by journal editors is whether research which has been conducted unethically should be published. The question is consonant with that of whether we should benefit from any of the research conducted so unethically in the Nazi concentration camps. It is more difficult to answer than the question of whether unethical research should deliberately be conducted so that others may benefit. That question, at least in its baldest theoretical form given here, should clearly be answered in the negative. But what about research which has already happened?

Some would argue that it is better that some good come out of unethical research than none, rather like the argument that fetal tissue should be used therapeutically, to ensure that some good comes out of an abortion. The counter argument to this is that such a stance will encourage bad practice in the future, giving house room to the idea that an action may be wrong in its content but it will be made right by its consequences. In any case, goes this side of the argument, if an action is wrong, then it is wrong, and no future outcome accidentally enjoyed by virtue of it makes it right. The debate is the classic one between consequentialist and deontological thinkers, in our terms the goal-based and the duty/right-based thinkers. Intuitively and idealistically I would like to believe that I would not knowingly benefit from another's harm. A different circumstance from medical research might elicit a different response from this, however. Suppose a Nazi tortures a Jewish freedom fighter who confesses that a bomb is placed outside some building. The Nazi tells me this information, and I know that my child is inside that building. Would I be wrong to save my child because the information was obtained unethically?

In the case of research, there is a difference between the status of research that has been conducted unethically according to goal-based standards, and that which has been unethical according to duty- or right-based standards. In the case of bad science (goal-based faults), the results cannot be extended to shed light on a new situation. In the case of deontologically bad (duty- or right-based faults) but methodologically good research the results may be relevant to a future situation. Suppose the research on the effects of the atmospheric conditions of an aeroplane on babies had shown that there is indeed a causal relationship between exposure to 15% oxygen and sudden infant death syndrome? However unethically the research had been conducted, that knowledge ought to be publicized, for the sake of future babies.

It is, I still contend, important to remain deeply intuitively uncomfortable with this situation. The usefulness of the results does not exonerate the unethical conduct of the research. Allowing good consequences to justify bad actions encourages bad actions. Therefore, the messy policy of journal editors, to publish research that is important scientifically but that has failed to meet duty- and right-based criteria, but to do so hedged around by commentaries, has, on balance, to be welcomed. The fact that it is difficult and uncomfortable, and satisfies no one completely, is a witness to our continued moral sensitivity and watchfulness. That is to be celebrated, not least because it ensures that attempts will continue to be made not to start research that is unethical. Better for the journal editors not to be faced with manuscripts of unethical research. Needless to say, there will always be debates, keeping researchers and research ethics committees busy, about the degree to which goal-, duty- or right-based concerns have to be compromised or outweigh each other before a research proposal becomes downright unethical.

Written consent

Written consent – the patient's signature on a piece of paper indicating her agreement to take part in a research project – may seem to represent one of the details of the consent procedure which has been finally established as a necessary detail and is therefore not open to question. The reason I want to discuss it here is because there is evidence that patients regard the practice of signing a consent form as a means of protecting the doctor, which is not what its purpose was supposed to be. I would argue that the signature on the piece of paper symbolizes the false worship of autonomy. It signifies a handing over of the moral responsibility for what follows to the patient and away from the doctor. The price of patient autonomy in this symbolism is the loss of the sense of being looked after by the doctor.

Empirical evidence that patients think their signature protects the doctor

The empirical evidence shows that patients think the signature on the consent form makes it a legal document absolving them of the right to make any claim against the doctor who treats them. Chee Saw et al. (1994) found this view in 62% of the patients in their trial. Dawes and Davison (1994), in a study of the success of the consent procedure in surgery for ear, nose and throat, stated: 'More than two thirds [of the study subjects] thought signing a consent form primarily signified agreement to undergo treatment and that it was a legal document; 54% thought there was an important medico-legal aspect'. When asked which of the following statements best reflected their attitude when signing the consent form, 14% thought it protected the doctor against being sued, while 90% thought they had to sign it. A study by Penman et al. (1984) found that 63% of patients receiving investigational chemotherapy said that the consent form played no part in their decision to accept treatment, saying that it was their trust in their doctor's guidance that was most important. A more recent study supported this finding (Mark and Spiro, 1990).

Consent as a separate, necessary procedure

The consent procedure, which involves offering adequate information and eliciting a voluntary response, is not covered by the signature on the piece of paper. Moreover, the consent procedure itself stands outside the doctor's responsibility for his patient which should be there whatever the patient has agreed to. These points were well put by a correspondent discussing the issue of consent to blood transfusion:

Inform[ing] patients adequately ... is exactly the factor that ensures that consent is both appropriate and valid, regardless of whether a formal consent form is signed by a patient in the presence of a healthcare professional ... The signature of a patient on a consent form does not mean that he or she assumes responsibility for the decision to give a transfusion: this remains with the doctor (Richardson and Jones, 1998).

In the *Sidaway* case the issue was whether valid consent had been obtained prior to an operation. Lord Scarman said, 'Mrs. Sidaway signed the usual consent form, in which she declared the nature and purpose of the operation had been explained to her'. But the case went through all the courts in an effort to establish what was really said to Mrs. Sidaway.

What, then, is the purpose of the signature? Is it to prove not to the law courts, but to those others who are tasked with checking on the researcher, that he is doing what he should be doing? How will research ethics committees know that any attention has been paid to consent if there is no signed consent form somewhere in existence? How will the Good Clinical Practice auditors (ICHGCP, 1997) know that the procedures for consent have been properly followed if there are no signed consent forms to look at? Yet it is within most people's experience to sign something they have not read, particularly if it is being held out by a (busy) doctor or a nurse, whom they believe has their best interests at heart.

The effect of the consent form on the research participant

The evidence points to the suspicion that, for a research participant, signing a form has the effect of making her doubt that her doctor is entirely happy about what he is about to do to her, so much so that she has to sign something saying she will not sue the doctor if it goes wrong, even though the form does not indicate as much. If the consent form were just a bureaucratic example of the increasingly regulated times then it would not matter quite so much. But it does not help the patient, and it does not help the consent process.

Concluding remarks

Under the general heading of right-based concerns consent has been identified as the most important moral claim. The obligation to obtain consent arises from the principle that no-one should be used merely as a means to an end but always also as an end in herself. That, I contended, is a moral principle which stands alone, not needing support from goal-based reasons of consequence, nor from duty-based reasons of not harming. It is simply the right that accrues to human beings. Of course, it can only accrue to human beings who have autonomy to exercise. The implications of this were discussed in Chapter Four. In this chapter the various ways in which the principle of consent is threatened were considered. They come in three guises, which approximate to the three moral approaches which have been the framework for this book. The right-based threats were found in a large amount of empirical evidence that the consent procedure does not work very well. Information is misunderstood, and people do not feel free or well enough to make voluntary decisions. In particular, there is a block about the meaning and implications of randomization. The apparent inability of many people to understand what random allocation is may be symptomatic of a refusal to believe that their doctor is so uncertain of what is best for them individually that he will prefer to toss a coin to allocate treatment. The objective, scientific arguments for randomization cannot easily be faulted, and many would objectively agree that if a valid result is to be reached, randomization is the best way. It is difficult for an individual to accept that for herself, however, because she knows that she is a peculiarly unique individual, different from every single other individual alive or dead. The paradox was nicely described by Professor Baum, who told a working party on informed consent that he had spoken to a patient about a clinical trial for which she was eligible. She had responded by asserting that she did not want to make the decision for herself, but wanted Baum to decide what was best for her. He said that he felt the best thing for her was to be in the trial, where she would have a 50% chance of receiving the best treatment. She said that she did not want to be in the trial. 'Which treatment would you prefer, then?' asked Baum. 'I don't know, you decide', was her response.

Duty-based threats to the principle of respect for autonomy show themselves more in theoretical arguments than in any empirical evidence that people will be adversely affected either by too much information, or by being required to decide for themselves what to do about their treatment. Particularly in the context of therapeutic research, where, it is argued, patients are receiving as good treatment as if they were being treated in the ordinary way, it should be left to the discretion of the researcher whether or not to seek consent. However, the difference between treatment and therapeutic research is the element of randomization, and as we have seen, that is a significant difference in the minds of patients. Unless she is explicitly told to the contrary, a patient will assume that her doctor has given her the treatment which her doctor (not a computer) has chosen for her, on the grounds that he believes it is the best treatment for her as an individual. Hence, not to tell patients about randomization, however difficult doing so might be, constitutes deceit.

The goal-based arguments against consent can be compelling, if good research is seriously under threat because of the consent requirement. Nevertheless, just as it would be wrong to conduct research which broke a goal-based rule by being badly designed, so would it be wrong to conduct research which broke a right-based rule by not seeking consent. The importance of respect for autonomy is too great to be easily overruled by consequentialism.

Finally, the practice of seeking written consent, a practice which has become standardized during the 1990s, was considered. It was argued that its value is very limited indeed, and that it may well do more harm than good, if the good we are seeking is a proper consent procedure. There is irony in the fact that the signed form neither protects the practitioner, nor does it allay patient fears. Its continued use seems irrational and counterproductive.

Confidentiality

Confidentiality is a right-based issue because it concerns the protection of personal information which, if it does not belong to the person, certainly does not belong to anyone else. Information which has been given in a clinical context should always be assumed to be confidential.

Should records-based or epidemiological research take place if it compromises patient autonomy?

Records-based research is typically conducted by epidemiologists, and involves looking only at patient records with no interaction with patients at all. As said in Chapter Four, the principle governing confidentiality in the medical context is that while consent to disclosure may be inferred if the disclosure is to those who are directly involved in the patient's health care, it cannot be inferred if the recipient of the information is not so involved. This is the situation of the records-based researcher. The results of the research may lead to improvements in health care which might eventually benefit the patients whose records are being scrutinized, but the intention is not to benefit those patients directly. Hence, this is non-therapeutic research being conducted without patient consent, using information which is personal to those patients. The numbers involved may be huge, and the researcher unlikely to know the patients. Indeed, the researcher is unlikely to be the slightest bit interested in who the patient is whose records he is examining: he will only be looking for what interests him, and that will not be any unfortunate medical secrets about the patient. These practical observations do not detract from the fact that for such research to take place, the principle of confidentiality has been violated. But, say epidemiologists, this research has to take place:

Probably every hazard we know of has required access to medical records, often with the details of the exposure kept in one place and the details of outcome in another, requiring a formal link between the two. The associations between taking oestrogens in pregnancy and cancer, ionising radiation and leukaemia, and use of oral contraceptives and venous thrombosis were all documented in this way. Recently, the risk of limb reduction defects associated with chorionic villus sampling in early pregnancy was identified through linking records. Such work can also provide reassuring information on the safety of medical procedures – for example, confirmation that amniocentesis does not cause clubfoot. The comparison of the results of blood tests from pregnant women with and without specified congenitally malformed fetuses has led to the development of antenatal screening tests. (Wald et al., 1994)

One solution to the problem of breaching confidentiality is to anonymize the records before the researcher sees them. This has serious resource implications (a goal-based problem), although it is possible. But in any case, the examples of the benefits of records-based research quoted above all depended upon the records being named so that they could be linked. Another solution would be to seek the consent of all the people whose records are involved. This, again, has such huge resource implications that much, if not all, records-based research would simply not be able to commence on that basis.

However, the right-based moral claim to privacy is strong, so much so that versions of the two solutions given above were threatened in European legislation, although they were in the end waived if the disclosure was for research purposes. When it looked like they would be made law, Wald and others (1994) argued strongly that such moves had to be resisted. They gave the examples listed above as arguments for being allowed to continue with their epidemiology, which are all goal-based, in that they seek to justify the breach of confidentiality by reference to the vast amount of good it has done. They further argue, using a sort of compromised right-based approach, that records were frequently shared already for the purposes of care of the patient, and that:

In practice, the duty of confidentiality is interpreted as applying not only to the doctor directly involved in the care of the patient but also to those with whom he or she judges the information may be shared; there is, in effect, a professional duty of collective confidentiality... Once the sense of sharing personal medical information among doctors – subject to a strict duty of collective confidentiality – is accepted, it becomes irrelevant whether the activity is for research, teaching, or care. The only relevant issue is to ensure that the collective confidentiality is secure and that no breach occurs that could in any way adversely affect the individuals concerned. (Wald et al., 1994)

The lack of distinction between the uses to which the records are being put is disingenuous. Of course it makes a difference: consent can be inferred, as I said, if the reason for disclosure is in the best interests of the patient; such an inference cannot be made otherwise.

It would seem that the conflict is a moral one: either the right-based demand for respect to privacy strictly interpreted wins, and such research, much needed, cannot take place; or the research is permitted to take place for goal-based reasons and the right-based claim is overridden. In the UK, guidelines from the Department of Health (1996) provide a fudge which nevertheless lets the goal-based view take the upper hand: they say that if a researcher has a contract with the National Health Service, and is therefore bound by the rules of confidentiality that all National Health Service personnel are bound by, and if the local research ethics committee agrees, then the researcher may have access to patient records without consent. The fudge provides a loophole: epidemiologists who wish to gain access to patient records but who have no National Health Service contract simply obtain a short-term contract. This does mean, of course, they must abide by rules of confidentiality.

Concluding remarks

The solution provided by the UK guidance is useful, since it allows epidemiologists to continue their work whilst at the same time emphasizing the importance of the confidentiality principle. That is the best that can be hoped for. The principle of confidentiality *is* important. But to rule out all epidemiological research automatically by making the principle absolute does not accord with commonsense (a good test for ethical decision making). It ignores the context, which is usually a mistake. By hedging the breach around with conditions, respect is paid to the principle without letting it become a dictator.

Summary and concluding remarks

This chapter has considered right-based issues as they arise in research on humans. The issues are those of consent and confidentiality. How the principle of respect for autonomy may come under threat from right-, duty- and goal-based perspectives has been considered, as has what threatens confidentiality, and how strong the arguments are for undermining it. Solutions have not been provided, but rather we have shown how it is possible for there to be disagreement about the ethics of a research project. By dividing up the different ethical concerns into three approaches we can see how a project can fulfil one but not necessarily all of them. Although the decision still has to be taken, if the approaches come into conflict, as to whether or not a research project should go ahead, the analysis by reference to the three approaches helps to clarify what, if anything, we are compromising by virtue of our decision. It also, importantly, retains the integrity of the different moral claims. By making explicit the fact that, for example, right-based morality has been waived in order to allow an epidemiological research project to happen, the issue has not been fudged but we have rather been clear about what we are doing. The task has also been given of demonstrating why the right-based principle should be subsumed in this particular case. Having to do that means having to take the principle seriously. That can help prevent unethical research through ignorance of the moral issues at stake.

9

A framework for ethical review: researchers, research ethics committees, and moral responsibility

Introduction

How well does the three-approaches system of ethics work in the context of research on humans? Three approaches to making moral decisions have been identified (following Botros): goal-based, duty-based and right-based. Goal-based morality is consequentialist, duty- and right-based morality are deontological. As they have been defined here, duty- and right-based morality consider the content of the action itself; the distinction between them is the way in which the rightness of the action is judged. Duty-based morality asks that the action be in accord with moral principles that are believed to be right regardless of the situation. Right-based morality, by contrast, considers the wishes and concerns of those affected by the action, not only in terms of whom the action will make happy and whom not, but also in terms of their views on the content of the action.

The three approaches combined

Although libraries of books have been written about versions of these three approaches, and indeed about other ways of thinking morally about actions, the three-approaches model works well for the purposes of considering the ethics of research on humans because it can form a framework for ethical review of research projects. Rather than try to decide which of the three approaches is the best one, I have found that all three approaches have their place in the decision-making process. Each is deficient in some way, but the deficiency is made up by the other two. Hence, the failure of goal-based morality to consider the content of the action which leads to greater happiness would mean that some morally abhorrent acts might be countenanced. Duty-based morality fills in the gap, because it asks that actions in general adhere to certain moral principles, among which would include not deliberately harming anyone when acting. On its own, duty-based morality can be blinkered, in that the moral principles do need to be applied intelligently in given contexts. Goal-based thinking provides the context: it identifies a goal and describes how it needs to achieve that goal. Duty-based morality, though, should not be put off by strident goal-based claims: however justified the research might seem in terms of its outcome, there are some research projects which are too risky to research subjects to be acceptable. The experiment with babies in 15% oxygen tents discussed in Chapter Seven was an example of that. At certain points, the duty-based moralist will argue that whatever the consequences, there are some things that should not be countenanced. For of course, unlike duty- and right-based morality, goal-based morality not only prohibits certain actions (which lead to a decrease in happiness), it also positively requires certain other actions. If an action *will* increase happiness, then it is morally wrong by goal-based standards not to do it. This argument can be used by researchers to justify what they do. The controlled trials which validate new treatments not only do not violate moral (goal-based) principles, they are also positively demanded by moral (goal-based) principles, because the consequences of a treatment not being properly validated are far worse than the consequences of its being validated (e.g. Wing, 1975). This is an argument that has to be taken seriously. The context of moral decision-making matters and the goals of a research project set that context. Ignoring the goal-based imperative by making duty- and right-based principles absolute creates a tyranny within which no one flourishes, just as making science and its pursuit an absolute creates a tyranny.

Typically, the duty-based concern will be with the harm to which the research participants will be exposed. Any harm from research should be justifiable and acceptable. In therapeutic research, the harm should be no greater than that which patient would expect if they were patients only and not research participants as well. The benefits they might expect from therapy should also be the same, as far as anyone can tell, in the research context as compared with the practice context. This requires strong equipoise, or a genuine balance of uncertainty about the efficacy of the comparative arms of the study. In non-therapeutic research, the duty-based moralist requires harm to be minimized for the research subjects who can expect no therapeutic benefit from participation.

Duty-based morality, as well as courting the danger of preventing clinicians from doing anything new and experimental, is also lacking in its consideration of the autonomy, or reasonableness, of the people most affected by the action itself. In the context of research, these are the research participants. The trust relationship between doctor and patient means that patients will assume that a doctor will not ask them to do things which are harmful. Therefore, doctors should ensure that in non-therapeutic research the risk is minimal. Nevertheless, doctors should also be wary of being overly paternalistic in their assessments of what procedures their patients would accept for the sake of others. Most human beings are capable of and want to think about whether what they are about to do is right or not. This is true of the researcher in a research project, but it is also crucially true of the research participants. The duty-based moralist may think she knows what is best for her research participants; but they may take a different view. Hence, the potential research participants need to be asked whether they are willing to take part in research, and whether they think that whatever they will have to face as research participants constitutes an acceptable risk or not. If a trial has satisfied goal-based requirements by aiming at a laudable goal, it has the potential to do good. Blocking it because of a fear on behalf of the potential research participants is not always a good idea. Those who will be exposed to the risk should be asked what they think.

Moreover, even if the duty-based moralist is entirely satisfied that the research is not exposing subjects to undue harm, for instance in the well-designed therapeutic research project, it is still wrong not to ask the subjects if they mind participating. Again, I have discussed suggestions, which are a mixture of goal- and duty-based, that if the research is aiming at a good goal, the researcher is in strong equipoise and the research participants will really be treated just as well, if not better, in a trial than otherwise, then they do not need to be consulted about whether they should take part or not. This viewpoint is an affront to persons who will thereby be used merely instrumentally. In any case, there may be all sorts of reasons particular to individuals why participating in a research project is unacceptable, however much good their doctors may think it will do them and future patients like them. So the moral necessity of seeking consent from subjects to participate in research, demanded by right-based morality, must be respected. The tendency of duty-based morality to speak on behalf of others is thus modified by right-based morality.

A framework to assist ethical review

The three-approaches framework can be translated into a series of questions, the consideration of which helps lead to a sound and reasonable analysis of the ethics of a proposed research project. They are offered in order of appearance, not in order of importance.

Goal-based questions

- What question is the research project addressing?
- Is the research aiming at a goal which is good and desirable?
- How will the research achieve that goal so that the results are reliable?
- How will the results of the research be disseminated?

Duty-based questions

- Are the procedures, which research participants will have to undergo for the trial to reach a successful conclusion, unacceptably risky?
- If therapeutic research, is there equipoise?
- If non-therapeutic research, are the risks greater than minimal?

Right-based questions

- Will consent will be sought from potential research subjects?
- What procedures to obtain consent will be followed?
- How will confidentiality be respected?

Resolving conflicts between the three approaches

Goal-based questions to set the context

When considering the ethics of any given research project we should begin by asking what question the research project is addressing. This sets the context for the moral analysis which follows. The next question is goal-based because it asks whether the question being investigated is important. Next comes the question of the way in which the question is going to be answered. This is, essentially, another context-setting rather than moral question, because all it does is to identify the appropriate research method for the type of question being asked, a morally neutral step. However, the way a research project is designed is crucial to its moral acceptability, since if it is not designed in such a way that the question will be answered, then it is a waste of all sorts of resources. Worse still, the answer may be wrong but believed, and it will then be the cause of wrong or bad practice being introduced into medical care. The fourth goal-based question is about the dissemination and assimilation of the results of the research. Again, the question is morally neutral but the answer is not. Research which never sees the light of day, particularly if it has been properly designed and has asked a question whose answer is worth knowing, is also a waste of all sorts of resources.

Goal-based and duty-based moral imperatives in conflict

Once these four questions are dealt with the research needs to be considered from a duty-based perspective. Is the research design, which has been decided is the right one for this research question, going to expose the research participants who have to adhere to it to undue risk of harm? Here is where the first signs of conflict can begin to show themselves. If the research is non-therapeutic, the duty-based thinker may have profound problems with any risk to the research participants, no matter how important the goals of the research may be. If there is a non-therapeutic research project with a very desirable goal but which exposes participants to harm, should it take place or not? This is the conflict between goal-based and duty-based morality. Goal-based morality says the research should happen; duty-based morality says not. If the goal-based moralist wins the argument, what harm might befall the research participants? If the duty-based moralist wins, what developments in medicine might thereby be curtailed?

If the research is therapeutic, equipoise is demanded by the duty-based thinker. Often this will be present in the design of the research with its different arms giving different treatments, all comparable. However, the goal-based argument for the need for placebo controls tips the balance against duty-based acceptability, for in placebo-controlled trials, as we saw, unless the standard treatment for the condition under research is in fact no treatment, strong equipoise is not present. Another dilemma emerges at the point of interaction between goal- and duty-based morality. The scientific merit of the placebo-controlled trial is very significantly greater than active-controlled trials in the eyes of many, so much so that the US Food and Drug Administration *requires* a placebo control unless the condition being treated is life-threatening or serious. The duty-based thinker balks at the fact that patients are not being treated equitably in a trial, that they have a chance of receiving no treatment, when had they been patients in the ordinary way they would have received some. The goal-based thinkers may seek to compromise themselves to the duty-based thinkers by restricting placebo-controlled trials to conditions which are not serious, as the FDA does, hence arguing that exposure to placebo would not cause outright harm. But, as one strident duty- (and right-) based thinker has put it, as far as the patient is concerned, she is ill enough to have sought treatment. Thus, in the eyes of at least one person, arguably the most interested and therefore the person whose opinion counts for most, placebo, when standard treatments exist, is not acceptable (Freedman et al., 1997b). Despite the FDA's requirements, the issue is not settled, and such a policy may produce a really unethical trial by duty-based standards because it potentially allows scientific rigour to override protection of individuals from harm.

Goal-based and right-based

The next, right-based, set of questions relates to the need to treat all the research participants as ends in themselves. Hence their consent must be sought and their confidentiality respected. In the case of any research project involving competent participants, whose private data will be protected from disclosure save with their agreement, these right-based requirements do not, on the face of it, conflict with goal- and duty-based requirements. However, some research projects' scientific validity depends upon research participants not knowing that they are subjects in a trial, such as the trial comparing different follow-up care for women having treatment for breast cancer discussed in Chapter Eight. In cases such as these, either the women's consent is not sought, or the research is useless. Either goal-based or right-based moral demands win out; they cannot both be fulfilled.

Another way in which goal- and right-based demands conflict is research which can only happen if patient confidentiality is breached. This is the situation with medical records research discussed in Chapter Eight. As we saw in that case, UK regulations (Department of Health, 1996) have come to a decision to allow the goal-based requirements to override the right-based ones, whilst taking into account the minimal level of insult and so not ignoring the right-based approach.

Duty-based and right-based

Right- and duty-based morality come into conflict when the duty-based concern for the welfare and well-being of the potential research participant will, in the eyes of the moral agent or researcher, be threatened by seeking consent to participate in a trial, and yet, as far as her (duty-based) eye can see, it would be most beneficial for her patient to go into his trial. The conflict between the duty-based concern for the patient's welfare and the right-based concern for his autonomy is given an added complication, and edge, by the goal-based problem that seeking consent reduces recruitment rates. In some cases it reduces them so much that trials have to be abandoned, which to the predominantly goal-based thinker is a tragedy of quite extreme dimensions, particularly as, to her mind, the patients who refused entry would have been treated as well if not better in the trial than outside it. Does autonomy have a price? Some would argue that it does not, as it is that which makes us human, and demands that we treat others as ends and not means. It is our recognition of a person's autonomy which makes us treat him or her as of equal worth to ourselves. It was the failure to recognize the inmates of the concentration camps as humans with autonomy, namely to dehumanize them and thus make them expendable, which made it possible for the Nazi doctors to do what they did. But even with such compelling arguments as these, the goal- and duty-based arguments should not be automatically overridden. For some people make foolish decisions. Although they do have that right, if their foolish decisions affect many other people, perhaps there is an argument for ignoring them, or preventing them. Some would say that clinical trials of important new treatments, put in jeopardy because patients do not know what is best for them, are examples of this. Others would disagree.

Goal-based and right-based again

A final conflict might be seen between right-based and goal-based demands when the subjects are incompetent and hence their consent cannot be sought. If a research project involving incompetent participants takes place, the goal-based approach has won. In a way it is a false hypothesis, however, since in the case of incompetent participants right-based morality has nothing to say, for consent cannot be sought, and it is confusing to argue as if it can. In these cases, the duty-based demands for protection become doubly important, and the right-based concerns for respecting patient confidentiality remain. I might argue that because the research participants cannot speak for themselves, duty-based concerns must always override goal-based ones. Whilst this seems intuitively right, I would still caution attempts to make hard and fast rules.

When the three approaches fail

The foregoing discussion has assumed that it is possible to answer the moral demands of each of the three approaches, even if it is not always possible to answer all three of them in any one research project. Cases discussed in Chapters Six to Eight have shown that it is questionable whether even this can be so. For although the goal-based thinker can identify goals of research, it is more often than not hard to decide just how important they are. Although she can define the methods needed to answer the research question, rarely will a research method answer it perfectly. The duty-based thinker can seek to protect research participants from foreseeable harm, but no one can protect them from unforeseeable harm. The right-based thinker can demand that consent be sought, but no one can guarantee that consent is actually obtained, however happy the patient is to sign the consent form.

Do these observations lead to the conclusion that medical research on humans is probably always immoral? I think if I answered that question in the affirmative I would have missed the point of the moral endeavour. For after all, we are not gods to determine our own and others' fate. We can try to do good, but we cannot be sure that we will succeed. What, in the end, the three approaches offer is a formulation of our motives for acting, not a recipe for their moral success. The three approaches ask that we seek to magnify the good (goal-based); that we are harmless (duty-based); and that we respect other people's autonomy (right-based).

This book has been addressed primarily to the moral agent, that is, the researcher, and not to the research ethics committee, although it is every bit as relevant to the latter as it is to the former. I hope it is relevant to everyone who is involved in medical research on humans, at whatever level and in whatever way. It is just that when it comes to making moral decisions about whether to act or not it is up to the agent of the action to make those decisions for him- or herself. We should not ask others to make those decisions for us. We can seek advice, and we can take and obey orders, but in the end we should only do so because we believe it is right. It may seem that we are driven to make certain decisions. Moral thinking is a way of waking up to the fact that how we act is up to us, and, therefore, since actions have consequences, we should do as much good as we possibly can. It is a way, in short, of becoming free and responsible, a choice which is available to every rational being. This book is addressed to researchers because it is up to them to take on the moral responsibility for the research on humans which they conduct. The three approaches are meant to help that process work intelligently. If there is an emotional commitment in researchers to the intentions the three approaches identify, they will be acting as morally as they can and are to be supported for that, whatever the success or otherwise of the enterprise.

Research ethics committees

Research Ethics Committees came into being partly because researchers were not, as far as those who were commenting on the situation could tell, behaving as well as they should, and partly because a shift in moral emphasis from goal- and duty-based thinking to right-based thinking, with which doctors had seemingly not kept up, meant that some sort of external pressure needed to be put on researchers to adopt a more right-based approach. More kindly, but more tellingly, the idea was to provide a means by which researchers could consult the views of those who were not so closely concerned with their research goals as they were, and so were in a better position to judge the ethics of what they were doing more fairly. This, although well meant and probably needed, held out the possibility of moving the moral responsibility for a research project one step away from the researcher herself and on to the shoulders of the research ethics committee which, in the end, has become not an advisory body but one which has positively to approve the ethics of any research on humans before it takes place. Whilst the work of research ethics committees has been really good, and their function very necessary, their creation and development into gatekeepers for research on humans has a sad inevitability about it. It is inevitable because, as will be shown, it is hard to see how things could have developed otherwise. It is sad because the keenness of moral thinking that I have tried to demonstrate is so essential in the researcher has had the edge taken off it by virtue of her having to consult – and follow – the views of others. I am not decrying such actions, but once rules are written most people tend not to think about why they take the form they do, and whether they are really good rules or not. The rules that now surround research on humans are commendable but they do detract from the researcher's sense of personal moral responsibility. In what follows the history of the establishment of research ethics committees in the UK is recounted to show what I mean. In the US, where the equivalent Institutional Review Boards were established by law from the start, the general point still applies, that ethics is more than merely obeying a pre-written code.

The Nuremberg Code

The 1946 Nuremberg Code (Annas and Grodin, 1992) was drawn up following the trials at Nuremberg of, among others, the Nazi doctors who had conducted research on concentration camp inmates with such chilling cruelty. The Code consists of ten principles to govern research on humans, the first of which is a categorical requirement that consent should be obtained before anyone becomes a research subject. This Code was, as far as the literature can tell us, largely ignored by researchers, perhaps because they thought that the Code was only for badly behaved doctors like those tried at Nuremberg. Moreover, the Code dealt only with non-therapeutic research. During the 1950s, then, research was conducted but not under any sort of ethical scrutiny apart from that of the doctors themselves. This was in keeping with attitudes generally, for the doctors would regard themselves as professionals bound by strict ethical principles, and their patients would simply do as they were told.

Pappworth's guinea pigs

During the 1960s, however, attitudes began to modify. One instigator of change from within the medical profession was Dr Maurice Pappworth. He was investigating and writing throughout the 1960s of abuses of medical privilege in the interests of research. In 1969 his book *Human Guinea Pigs* was published. It begins with the following accusation:

For several years a few doctors in this country and in America have been trying to bring to the attention of their fellows a disturbing aspect of what have become common practices in medical research. These practices concern experiments made chiefly on hospital patients, and the aspect of them which is disturbing is the ethical one. In their zeal to extend the frontiers of medical knowledge, many clinicians appear temporarily to have lost sight of the fact that the subjects of their experiments are in all cases individuals with common rights and in most cases sick people hoping to be cured. As a result it has become a common occurrence for the investigator to take risks with patients of which those patients are not fully aware, or not aware at all, and to which they would not consent if there were aware; to subject them to mental and physical distress which is in no way necessitated by, and has no connexion with, the treatment of the disease from which they are suffering; and in some cases deliberately to retard the recovery from that disease so that investigation of a particular condition can be extended. (Pappworth, 1969)

His book describes the procedures of hundreds of experiments which bear out this observation. His sources of information were not difficult to find: they were chiefly articles published in the medical press. All he did, duty-based fashion, was to describe the methods, adopted in the research in order to gain the answer, from the point of view of the procedures which the patients would actually have undergone.

Sir Austin Bradford-Hill and Mrs Hodgson

In the lay public, an organization called the Patients' Association was beginning to make concerned noises. These were first prompted by some of the points raised in a lecture given by Sir Austin Bradford-Hill, a renowned medical statistician. He was speaking about the dangers of trying to codify ethics and make rules that apply for all time to research on humans. Some of his observations were prophetic, and these will be returned to later. Here, however, I reproduce the point that really irked Mrs Hodgson, chairman of the Patients' Association:

Personally, and speaking as a patient, I have no doubt whatever that there are circumstances in which the patient's consent to taking part in a controlled trial should be sought. I have equally no doubt that there are circumstances in which it need not – and even should not – be sought... Surely it is often quite impossible to tell ill-educated and sick persons the pros and cons of a new and unknown treatment versus the orthodox and known? And in fact, of course one does not know ... Can you describe that situation to a patient so that he does not lose confidence in you – the essence of the doctor/patient relationship – and in such a way that he fully understands and can therefore give an *understanding* consent to his inclusion in the trial? In my opinion nothing less is of value. Just to ask the patient does he mind if you try some new tablets on him does nothing, I suggest, to meet the problem ... If the patient cannot really grasp the whole situation, or without upsetting his faith in your judgement cannot be made to grasp it, then in my opinion the ethical decision still lies with the doctor, whether or not it is proper to exhibit, or withhold a treatment.

Three months later, an editorial in the *British Medical Journal* responded:

By his remarks about *not* telling patients of the whys and wherefores of an experiment, Sir Austin has attracted the attention of Mrs. Helen Hodgson, chairman of the Patients' Association, who in the *British Medical Journal* of May 18 sharply challenged him. Mrs. Hodgson, according to an article in the *Times* (June 17) headed 'Now a Voice for the Patient', is moving forward with some determination. A questionary is being sent out to members of the Patients' Association which says this: 'Clinical trials are obviously going on, and on a big scale. Patients are not told if they are receiving new or orthodox treatment. I maintain that they should be told. I think it begs the

question to say that it is difficult to explain these things to ignorant and sick people.'
We agree with Mrs. Hodgson. (*British Medical Journal*, 1963)

The Medical Research Council, the World Medical Association and the Royal College of Physicians

The medical profession, through its professional bodies, had not been entire-ly idle during this time. The Medical Research Council issued a statement in its report for the year 1962–63, entitled 'Responsibility in investigations in institutions' (Medical Research Council, 1964). This gave clear ethical prin-ciples that should govern research involving human subjects. The World Medical Association drew up the Declaration of Helsinki in 1964, also giving principles for research on humans, against the production of which Sir Austin Bradford-Hill was arguing in his 1963 lecture. Most effective of all, however, was the report issued by the Royal College of Physicians in 1967 to boards of governors, medical school councils and hospital management committees or equivalent bodies in non-medical institutions, and subse-quently endorsed by the Ministry of Health (1968). This Report quoted the Surgeon-General of the United States who, in 1966, had called upon the institutions which were state funded to take full responsibility for the re-search carried out in them. The College of Physicians Report said that medical institutions had a responsibility for ensuring that all clinical investi-gations carried out within their hospitals were ethical and conducted with the optimum technical skill and precautions for safety. The Report then states:

This responsibility would be discharged if in medical institutions where clinical investigation is carried out, it were ensured that all projects were approved by a *group of doctors* [my italics] including those experienced in clinical investigation. This group should satisfy itself of the ethics of all proposed investigations. (Royal College of Physicians, 1967)

The Ministry of Health

The endorsing Health Notice from the Ministry of Health issued the follow-ing year was sent to regional and area health authorities and to boards of governors, asking them to set up these advisory groups. Prototype research ethics committees were born.

The growth of research ethics committees' power

Until 1991 not every District Health Authority had a research ethics commit-tee, and until 1991 clear and detailed guidance was not forthcoming from the government as to how these committees should function, who should sit on them, and what the ethical criteria were against which to judge the research proposals being put before them (Foster, 1997b). But the authority of research ethics committees had grown. They began as advisory bodies, offering an independent view of the ethics of research proposals. For their function to be recognized and used by sometimes reluctant doctors, they had to have some authority, which meant that it needed to become mandatory to consult them. During the period from 1968 to 1991 no new legislation was proposed, as it had been in the United States from the beginning, but custom and practice required that if research was to take place on human subjects within the NHS, then research ethics committees had to be involved. What if a research ethics committee gave a view with which a researcher disagreed? For the research ethics committee's function to have any meaning, the committee had to have the final word. Advice changed to approval, and research ethics committees' authority strengthened.

The importance of the issues research ethics committees were considering, albeit not well defined during this period, was recognized by the editors of medical journals and those who funded or commissioned research. Over time it became a rule that a good journal would not publish a researcher's findings if her project had not first been approved by a research ethics committee. Those who awarded funds required ethical approval prior to granting support. The pharmaceutical industry required its researchers to obtain ethical approval; and in 1991 the (more) formal establishment of Local Research Ethics Committees (Department of Health, 1991) led to a move by the industry to seek approval from every local committee rather than a central one, as had hitherto been the practice for multi-centre trials. A trial was deemed to be ethical if it had been approved by a local research ethics committee; not otherwise. The differing interpretations of what constituted ethical research that had developed within committees around the country meant that local committees often came to different decisions about research which they had to approve. When the research was multi-centre this led to major logistical difficulties as the same trial would be judged differently around the country.

Multi-centre research ethics committees

Rather than ask the researcher to judge which were the right opinions, which was obviously inappropriate by this stage, the solution was to create a new set of committees, called Multi-centre Research Ethics Committees, which were to approve the ethics of multi-centre research, with local committees retaining the right to veto research in their patches for local reasons (Department of Health, 1997). This structure is reflected in proposed European legislation on the conduct of clinical trials.

'Who guards the guardians?'

One of the problems research ethics committees face is that although they can approve or disapprove the research proposal that the researcher puts before them, they cannot know that what they are shown is what actually takes place without actually being there. Some committees are setting themselves up as auditors to ensure that researchers do what the committees agreed they could do (Berry, 1997; Smith et al., 1997). Concerns of a similar nature are now being expressed about what happens in research ethics committees' meetings, where members may be making all sorts of mistaken judgements due to lack of understanding of the research they have to review (Foster and Holley, 1998). Without actually watching the committees in session we could not know. Some researchers regard the fact that a number of different committees, reviewing the same research project, come to different conclusions about it, to be proof that some committees are not working properly (Harries et al., 1994; Hotopf et al., 1995; Penn and Steer, 1995; Ahmed and Nicholson, 1996). The pharmaceutical industry, required by regulatory authorities to prove that it has conducted its research in an exemplary manner, needs to be sure that the research ethics committees which approve its research are functioning properly. In the United States, auditors from the FDA patrol committees and this may start to happen in the UK before too long. At some point a question will be raised as to whether the auditors are doing their work properly.

The point of telling the story of research ethics committees is not to undermine their sterling work, which has been undertaken in often extremely difficult circumstances for thirty years. I cannot praise the endeavour highly enough, because it has always been in support of the good. It is rather to emphasize that no amount of regulation, auditing or public accountability can detract from the fact that people are morally responsible for their own actions. The 'seen to be ethical' part of the ideal 'be ethical and be seen to be ethical', which is often invoked in the context of research on humans, is laudable, and the attempts that research ethics committees have made to make it meaningful are even more laudable. However, appearances can be deceptive, whereas everyone knows what she/he is up to individually. No one can hide from him- or herself.

Bradford-Hill's prophecy

Bradford-Hill had some unfortunate views about consent, which were at least partly responsible for the development of the regulatory system now used to govern medical research on humans. It is ironic that, in seeking to show the dangers of regulating research, he helped to bring about the very regulation he was keen to avoid. For the main message of his lecture was that once written regulations appear, no matter how much their status is said to be advisory rather than binding, they become the yardstick against which actions are measured, and ultimately the law's reference point, should there need to be one. In the end, he said, the Declaration of Helsinki, and other guidelines which follow, will not help a researcher conduct his research ethically, they will be the rules by which he is bound. The mark of advice is that it is followed freely, and can be ignored. The Declaration of Helsinki, should it be drawn up, would not long remain with that uncertain status. And, of course, Bradford-Hill was right. By virtue of the regulatory system we have for research on humans, the first step of which was the Declaration of Helsinki, the reason researchers conduct the research in the way they do is because they run the risk of working outside the law if they do not. That, at any rate, is the threat that calls researchers to order and gives research ethics committees the power they wield.

Conclusion

This legalism is a far cry from the project of this book, which is to provide researchers with the tools they need to be able to discern an ethical approach to their research. I would urge you to conduct a proper moral analysis using the framework for ethical review that I have offered, rather than to refer to rules which cannot anticipate every new situation. If you do use the framework it will be possible to demonstrate that your decision was made on a sound and reasonable basis, taking all the necessary factors into account. That, in the end, is what matters most.

References

ABPI (Association of the British Pharmaceutical Industry) (1991). Guidelines for safe laboratory practice. In Foster, C. (ed.) *Manual for Research Ethics Committees*, 5th edn, 1997. London: King's College.

Ahmed, A.H. and Nicholson, K.G. (1996). Delays and diversity in the practice of local research ethics committees. *Journal of Medical Ethics* **22**: 263–6.

Annas, G.J. and Grodin, M.A. (1992). *The Nazi Doctors and the Nuremberg Code.* New York, Oxford: Oxford University Press.

Aquinas, T. (*c.* 1264) *Summa Contra Gentiles.* transl. Vernon J. Bourke (1975). London: University of Notre Dame Press; New York: Doubleday.

Aspinall, R.L. and Goodman, N. (1995). Denial of effective treatment and poor quality of clinical information in placebo controlled trials of ondansetron for postoperative nausea and vomiting: a review of published trials. *British Medical Journal*, **311**: 844–6.

Baum, M. (1986). Do we need informed consent? *The Lancet*, October 18, **2**(8512): 911–12.

Baum, M. (1993). New approach for recruitment into randomised controlled trials. *The Lancet*, **341**: 812–13.

Bentham, J. (1789). *An Introduction to the Principles of Morals and Legislation.* In Warnock, M. (ed.) (1962). *Utilitarianism*, pp. 33–77. Glasgow: William Collins Sons and Co.

Berry, J. (1997). Local research ethics committees can audit ethical standards in research. *Journal of Medical Ethics*, **23**: 379–81.

Bhopal, R.S. and Tonks, A. (1994) The role of letters in reviewing research. *British Medical Journal*, **308**: 1582–3.

Black, D. (1998). The limitations of evidence. *Journal of the Royal College of Physicians*, **32**(1): 23–6.

Botros. S. (1992). Ethics in medical research: uncovering the conflicting approaches. In Foster, C. (ed.) *Manual for Research Ethics Committees*, 5th edn, 1997, vol. I, pp. iv, 1–10. London: King's College.

Boyd, R. (1998). A view from the man in the seat opposite. *British Medical Journal*, **317**: 410.

Bradford-Hill, A. (1963). Marc Daniels Lecture: Medical ethics and controlled trials. *British Medical Journal*, April 20: 1043–9.

Brewin, T.B. (1993). Logic and magic in mainstream and fringe medicine. *Journal of the Royal Society of Medicine*, **86**: 721–3.

British Medical Journal. (1963). Ethics of human experimentation (editorial). July 6, 5248–9.

British Medical Journal. (1983). Informed consent: ethical, legal and medical implications for doctors and patients who participate in randomised clinical trials (editorial). **286**: 1117–21.

British Paediatric Association. (1992). Guidelines for research on children. In Foster, C. (ed.) *Manual for Research Ethics Committees.* 5th edn, 1997, vol. II (27), pp. 1–24. London: King's College.

Britten, N. (1995). Qualitative interviews in medical research. *British Medical Journal,* **311**: 251–3.

Cairns, J.A., Gent, M., Singer, J. (1985). Aspirin, sulfinpyrazone, or both in unstable angina. *New England Journal of Medicine,* **313**: 1369–75.

Cassileth, B.R., Zupkis, R.V., Sutton-Smith, K. and March, V. (1980). Informed consent: why are its goals imperfectly realised? *New England Journal of Medicine,* **302**: 896–900.

Chalmers, I. (1994). Public involvement in research to assess the effects of healthcare. Paper presented to the Harveran Society, 12 January, 1994.

Chalmers, I. (1995). What do I want from health research and researchers when I am a patient? *British Medical Journal,* **316**: 1315–18.

Chee Saw, K., Wood, A.M., Murphy, K., Parry, J.R.W. and Hartfall, W.G. (1994). Informed consent: an evaluation of patients' understanding and opinion (with respect to the operation of transurethral resection of prostate). *Journal of the Royal Society of Medicine,* **87**: 143–4.

Ciociola, A.A., Webb, D.D. and McSorley, D.J. (1996). The continued use of placebo-controlled trials in the study of peptic ulcer disease: a sponsor perspective. *Drug Information Journal,* **30**: 433–9.

Collier, J. (1995). Confusion over the use of placebos in clinical trials. *British Medical Journal,* **311**: 821–2.

Collins, R., Doll, R. and Peto, R. (1992). Ethics of clinical trials. In Williams, C.J. (ed.) *Introducing New Treatments for Cancer: Practical, Ethical and Legal Problems.* Chichester: Wiley and Sons.

Darragh, A., Kenny, M., Lambe, R. and Brick, I. (1985). Sudden death of a volunteer. *The Lancet,* January 12th, pp. 93–4.

Dawes, P.J.D. and Davison, P. (1994). Informed consent: what do patients want to know? *Monash Bioethics Review,* **13**(4): 20–6.

Department of Health. (1991). *Local Research Ethics Committees.* HSG(91)5. London: HMSO.

Department of Health. (1996). *The Protection and Use of Patient Information.* HSG(96)18. London: HMSO.

Department of Health. (1997). *The Ethical Review of Multi-centre Research.* HSG(97)23. London: HMSO.

Dodds, E.C., Goldenberg, L., Lawson, W. and Robinson, R. (1938). Estrogenic activity of certain synthetic compounds. *Nature,* **141**: 247–8.

Dworkin, R. (1977). *Taking Rights Seriously.* London: Gerald Duckworth and Co. Ltd.

Easterbrook, P.J., Berlin, J.A., Gopalan R. and Matthews, D.R. (1991). Publication bias in clinical research. *Lancet,* **337**: 867–72.

Food, Drug and Cosmetic Act of 1938, 52 Stat. 1040, 21 U.S.C. paragraphs 301 et seq. at paragraph 505 (d) (as amended 1962).

Foster, C. 1996. Commentary: the ethics of clinical research without patients' consent. *British Medical Journal,* **312**: 817.

Foster, C. (ed.) (1997) *Manual for Research Ethics Committees,* 5th edn. King's College, London.

Foster, C. (1998). Research Ethics Committees. In Chadwick, R. (ed.) *Encyclopaedia of Applied Ethics,* vol. 3, pp. 845–52. San Diego: Academic Press, Inc.

Foster, C. and Holley, S. (1998). Ethical review of multi-centre research: a survey of multi-centre researchers in the South Thames region. *Journal of the Royal College of Physicians of London,* **32**(3): 242–5

Freedman, B., Weijer, C. and Cranley Grass, K. (1997a). Placebo orthodoxy in clinical research I: empirical and methodological myths. *Monash Bioethics Review,* **16**(4): 12–26.

Freedman, B., Weijer, C. and Cranley Grass, K. (1997b). Placebo orthodoxy in clinical research II: ethical, legal and regulatory myths. *Monash Bioethics Review,* **17**(1): 10–22.

Garnham, J.C. (1975). Some observations on informed consent in therapeutic research. *Journal of Medical Ethics,* **1**: 138–45.

Gillick v West Norfolk and Wisbech Area Health Authority [1986] AC 112, 169, 186, 188–89, 195, 201.

Goodman, N., Cooper, G.M., Malins, A.R. and Prys-Roberts, C. (1984). The validity of informed consent in a clinical study. *Anaesthesia,* **39**: 911–16.

Grubb, A. (1992). The law relating to consent. In Foster, C. (ed.) *Manual for Research Ethics Committees,* 5th edn, 1997, vol. I, pp. ii, 17–21. London: King's College.

Hare, R.M. (1986). Utilitarianism. In Macquarrie, J. and Childress, J. (eds.) *A New Dictionary of Christian Ethics,* pp. 640–3. London: S.C.M. Press, Ltd.

Harper, W. (1998). The role of futility judgements in improperly limiting the scope of clinical research. *Journal of Medical Ethics,* **24**(5): 308–13.

Harries, U.J., Fentem, P.H., Tuxworth, W. and Hoinville, W. (1994). Local research ethics committees: widely differing responses to a national survey protocol. *Journal of the Royal College of Physicians of London,* **28**: 150–4.

Hart, H.L.A. (1973). Bentham on legal rights. In Simpson, A.W.B. (ed.) *Oxford Essays on Jurisprudence,* second series, pp. 171–201. Oxford: Oxford University Press.

Harth, S.C. and Thong, Y.H. (1990). Sociodemographic and motivational characteristics of parents who volunteer their children for clinical research: a controlled study. *British Medical Journal,* **300**: 1372–5.

Hatch, E.E., Palmer, J.R., Titus-Ernstoff, L., et al. (1998). Cancer risk in women exposed to diethylstilbestrol in utero. *Journal of the American Medical Association,* **280**: 630–4.

Herxheimer, A. (1993). Publishing the results of sponsored clinical research. *British Medical Journal,* **307**: 1296–7.

HFEA/HGAC. (1998). *Cloning issues in reproduction, science and medicine.* London: Department of Trade and Industry.

Holtzman, N.A., Faden, R., Chwalow, A.J. and Horn, S.D. (1983). Effects of informed parental consent on mothers' knowledge of newborn screening.

Pediatrics, **72(6)**: 807–12.

Hotopf, M., Wessely, S. and Norman, N. (1995). Are ethical committees reliable? *Journal of the Royal Society of Medicine,* **88**: 31–5.

Hoy, A.M. (1985). Breaking bad news to patients. *British Journal of Hospital Medicine,* August, 96–9.

Hughes, V. (1998). Commentary: ethical approval of study was warranted. *British Medical Journal,* **317**: 892–3.

Hurwitz, B. (1998). *Clinical Guidelines and the Law.* Oxford: Radcliffe Medical Press.

International Conference on Harmonisation Good Clinical Practice (ICHGCP) (1997). International conference on harmonisation of technical requirements for registration of pharmaceuticals for human use. *Guidelines for good clinical practice.* Relevant excerpts can be found in Foster, C. (ed.) *Manual for Research Ethics Committees,* 5th edn, vol. II(2), pp. 1–30. London: King's College.

Jones, B., Jarvis, P., Lewis, J.A. and Ebbutt, A.F. (1996). Trials to assess equivalence: the importance of rigorous methods. *British Medical Journal,* **313**: 36–9.

Jones, J. and Hunter, D. (1995). Consensus methods for medical and health services research. *British Medical Journal,* **311**: 376–80.

Jones, R. (1995). Why do qualitative research? *British Medical Journal,* **311**: 2–3.

Kanis, J.A. and Bergmann, J.F. (1993). Full consent may bias outcome of trials (letter). *British Medical Journal,* **307**: 1497.

Kant, I. (1785). *Fundamental Principles of the Metaphysic of Morals.* Translated by Abbott, T.K. (1988). New York: Prometheus Books.

Kant, I. (1787). *Critique of Pure Reason.* Translated by Kemp Smith, N. (1978). London: Macmillan.

Keen, J. and Packwood, T. (1995). Case study evaluation. *British Medical Journal,* **311**: 444–6.

Kennedy, I.M. (1988). *Treat Me Right.* Oxford: Clarendon Paperbacks.

Kerridge, I., Lowe, M. and Henry, D. (1998). Ethics and evidence-based medicine. *British Medical Journal,* **316**: 1151–3.

Kerrigan, D.D., Thevasagayam, R.S., Woods, T.O. et al. (1993). Who's afraid of informed consent? *British Medical Journal,* **306**: 298–300.

King, J. (1986). Informed Consent. *Institute of Medical Ethics Bulletin,* Supplement no. 3 (stand alone publication). London: Institute of Medical Ethics.

Kitzinger, J. (1995). Introducing focus groups. *British Medical Journal,* **311**: 299–302.

Lancet editorial. (1993). Clinical trials and clinical practice. *Lancet.* 1993, **342**: 877–8.

Langman, M.J.S. (1997). Homeopathy trials: reason for good ones but are they warranted? *The Lancet.* 1997, **350**: 825.

Leeb, D., Bowers, D. and Lynch, J.B. (1976). Observations on the myth of 'informed consent'. *Plastic and Reconstruction Surgery.* 1976, **58(3)**: 280–2.

Lehrer, S. (1979). *Explorers of the Body.* Garden City, New York: Doubleday and Co. Ltd.

Ley, P. (1979). Memory for medical information. *British Journal of Social and Clinical Psychology.* 1979, **18**: 245–55.

Linde, K., Clausius, N., Ramirez, G., et al. (1997). Are the clinical effects of homeopathy placebo effects? A meta-analysis of placebo-controlled trials. *Lancet,* 350 (9081): 834–8.

MacRae, K. (1996). Clinical research statistics: some definitions. In Foster, C. (ed.) *Manual for Research Ethics Committees.* 5th edition, 1997, vol. I, pp. ii, 7. London: King's College.

Mark, J.S. and Spiro, H. (1990). Informed consent for colonoscopy: a prospective study. *Archives of Internal Medicine.* 1990, **150**: 777–80.

Marx, K. (1843). On the Jewish Question. In *Early Writings.* Transl. Rodney Livingstone and Gregor Benton (1973), pp. 211–41. London: Harmondsworth. (Can also be found in any collection of Marx's early writings.)

Mays, N. and Pope, C. (1995). Observational methods in health care settings. *British Medical Journal.* 1995, **311**: 182–4.

McArdle, J.M.C., George, W.D., McArdle, C.S. et al. 1996. Psychological support for patients undergoing breast cancer surgery: a randomised study. *British Medical Journal.* 1996, **312**: 813–17.

McBride, G. (1994). Phase one trials can exploit terminally ill patients. *British Medical Journal,* **308**: 679–80.

McDaniel Hutson, M. and Blaha, J.D. (1991). Patients recall of pre-operative instruction for informed consent for an operation. *Journal of Bone Joint Surgery (America),* **73**(a): 160–2.

Medical Research Council. (1964). Responsibility in investigations on human subjects. In *Report for the Year 1962–3,* pp. 21–5. London: HMSO (Cmnd 2382).

Ministry of Health. (1968). *Supervision of the Ethics of Clinical Trial Investigations.* HM(68)33. London: HMSO.

Noller, K.L. and Fish, C.R. (1974). Diethylstilbestrol usage: its interesting past, important present, and questionable future. *Medical Clinician of North America.* **58**: 739–810.

Nuremberg Trials (1946). Transcript of proceedings. In Kennedy, I. and Grubb, A. (1995) *Medical Law, Text and Materials,* pp. 1011–24. London: Butterworths.

Pappworth, M. (1969). *Human Guinea Pigs.* London: Routledge and Kegan Paul.

Parkins, K.J., Poets, C.F., O'Brien, L.M., Stebbens, V.A. and Southall, D.P. (1998a). Effect of exposure to 15% oxygen on breathing patterns and oxygen saturation in infants: interventional study. *British Medical Journal,* **316**: 887–94.

Parkins, K.J., Poets, C.F., O'Brien, L.M., Stebbens, V.A. and Southall, D.P. (1998b). Authors' reply. *British Medical Journal,* **316**: 893–4.

Penman, D.T., Holland, J.C., Bahna, G.F. et al. (1984). Informed consent for investigational chemotherapy: patients' and physicians' perceptions. *Americal Journal of Clinical Oncology,* **2**: 849–55.

Penn, Z.J. and Steer, P.J. (1995). Local research ethics committees: hindrance or help? *British Journal of Obstetrics and Gynaecology,* **102**: 1–2.

Pieters, T. (1998). Marketing medicines through randomised controlled trials: the case of interferon. *British Medical Journal,* **317**: 1231–3.

Platt, R. (1972). *Private and Controversial.* London: Cassell and Co.

Popper, K.R. (1959) *The Logic of Scientific Discovery.* London: Routledge and Kegan Paul.

President's Commission for the study of ethical problems in medicine and biomedical and behavioral research. (1983). *The Law of Informed Consent in making Health Care Decisions,* vol 3. Washington DC: Government Printing Office.

Reilly, D., Taylor, M., Beattie, N.G.M., et al. (1994). Is evidence for homeopathy reproducible? *The Lancet,* **344**: 1601–6.

Richardson, N.G.B. and Jones, P.M. (1998). Responsibility for decision to give transfusion remains with doctor, not patient (letter). *British Medical Journal,* **316**: 779–10.

Roberts, I. (1998). An amnesty for unpublished trials. *British Medical Journal,* **317**: 763–4.

Rothstein, J. (1995). Attending to transitions: a medical student's encounter with transplantation. *Bulletin of Medical Ethics.* November: 13–19.

Royal College of Physicians. (1967). *Supervision of the Ethics of Clinical Research Investigations in Institutions.* London: Royal College of Physicians.

Sackett, D.L. and Wennberg, J.E. (1997). Choosing the best research design for each question. *British Medical Journal,* **315**: 1636.

Savulescu, J. (1998). Commentary: safety of participants in non-therapeutic research must be ensured. *British Medical Journal,* **316**: 891–2.

Scarmen, Lord Justice. (1986). Consent, communication and responsibility. *Journal of the Royal Society of Medicine,* **79**: 697–8.

Scott, J., Weir, D.G. and Kirke, P.N. (1994). Prevention of neural tube defects with folic acid a success but ... *Queens Journal of Medicine,* **87**: 705–7.

Sidaway v. Royal Bethlem Hospital Governors. [1985] 1 AC 871.

Simes, R.J., Tattersall, M.H.N., Coates, A.S., et al. (1986). Randomised comparison of procedures for obtaining informed consent in clinical trials of treatment for cancer. *British Medical Journal,* **293**: 1065–8.

Slevin, M.L., Stubbs, L., Plant, H.J., et al. (1990). Attitudes to chemotherapy: comparing views of patients with cancer with those of doctors, nurses and general public. *British Medical Journal,* **300**: 1458–60.

Smith, T., Moore, E.J.H. and Tunstall-Pedoe, H. (1997). Review by a local medical research ethics committee of the conduct of approved research projects, by examination of patients' case notes, consent forms, and research records, and by interview. *British Medical Journal,* **314**: 1588–90.

Snowdon, C., Garcia, J. and Elbourne, D. (1997). Making sense of randomisation: responses of parents of critically ill babies to random allocation of treatment in a clinical trial. *Social Science and Medicine* **45**(9): 1337–55.

Stacey, M. (1991). The potential of social science for complementary medicine – some introductory reflections. *Complementary Medicine Research,* **5**: 183–6.

Sutherland, H.J., Lockwood, G.A. and Till, J.E. (1990). Are we getting informed consent from patients with cancer? *Journal of the Royal Society of Medicine,* **83**: 439–43.

Taylor, K.M., Margolese, R.G. and Soskolne, C.L. (1984). Physicians' reasons for not entering patients into a randomised clinical trial of surgery for breast cancer. *New England Journal of Medicine,* **310**: 1363–7.

Temple, R. (1996). Problems in interpreting active control equivalence trials. *Accountability in Research,* **4**: 267–75.

Thorogood, M. (1996). Observational research: some definitions. In Foster, C. (ed.) *Manual for Research Ethics Committees,* 5th edn, 1997, vol. I, pp. ii, 8. London: King's College.

Tobias, J.S. and Souhami, R.L. (1993). Fully informed consent can be needlessly cruel. *British Medical Journal*, **307**: 1199–201.

Tramer, M., Reynolds, D.J.M., Moore, R.A. and McQuay, H.J. (1998). When placebo controlled trials are essential and equivalence trials are inadequate. *British Medical Journal*, **317**: 875–80.

Vandenbroucke, J.P. (1997). Homeopathy trials: going nowhere. *The Lancet*, **350**: 24.

Wald, N., Law, M., Meade, T. et al. (1994). Use of personal medical records for research purposes. *British Medical Journal*, **309**: 1422–4.

Waldron, J. (ed.) (1995). *Theories of Rights*. Oxford: Oxford University Press.

Wallace, L. (1984). Psychological preparation as a method of reducing the stress of surgery. *Journal of Human Stress*, Summer: 62–77.

Wallace, L. (1986). Informed consent to elective surgery: the 'therapeutic value'? *Social Science and Medicine*, **22**(1): 29–33.

Walsh, P. (1998). Commentary: doctors can never have a moral holiday. *British Medical Journal*, **316**: 1517.

Walsworth-Bell, J.P. (1993). Doctors should admit uncertainty (letter). *British Medical Journal*, **307**: 1495.

Watson, N. and Wyld, P.J. (1992). The importance of general practitioner information in selection of volunteers for clinical trials. *British Journal of Clinical Pharmacology*, **33**: 197–9.

Weiss, R.A. (1998). Xenotransplantation. *British Medical Journal*, **317**: 931–4.

Williams, B. (1993). *Morality*. Cambridge: Cambridge University Press.

Wing, J.K. (1975). The ethics of clinical trials. *Journal of Medical Ethics*, **1**: 174–5.

Woodward, W.E. (1979). Informed consent of volunteers: a direct measurement of comprehension and retention of information. *Clinical Research*, **27**: 248–52.

World Medical Association. (1996). *Declaration of Helsinki*. Latest version: South Africa.

Wyatt, J.C., Paterson-Brown, S., Johanson, R., et al. (1998). Randomised trial of educational visits to enhance use of systematic reviews in 25 obstetric units. *British Medical Journal*, **315**: 1041–6.

Yunus, M. (with Jolis, A.) (1998). *Banker to the Poor*. London: Aurum Press, Ltd.

Index